REFLECTIONS of the
MOON on WATER

HEALING

WOMEN'S

BODIES

AND MINDS

THROUGH

TRADITIONAL

CHINESE

WISDOM

REFLECTIONS
of the
MOON on WATER

Xiaolan Zhao, CMD

with KANAE KINOSHITA

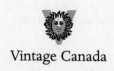

Vintage Canada

VINTAGE CANADA EDITION, 2007
Copyright © 2006 Xiaolan Zhao

Published in Canada by Vintage Canada, a division of Random House of Canada Limited, Toronto, in 2007. Originally published in hardcover in Canada by Random House Canada, a division of Random House of Canada Limited, Toronto, in 2006. Distributed by Random House of Canada Limited, Toronto.

Vintage Canada and colophon are registered trademarks of Random House of Canada Limited. Random House Canada and colophon are trademarks.

www.randomhouse.ca

Note: The information in this book is intended as complementary and is not designed to take the place of medical care. You should consult a physician before embarking on any treatment plan.

All patients' names in this book have been changed to protect their privacy.

Library and Archives Canada Cataloguing in Publication

Zhao, Xiaolan
          Reflections of the moon on water : healing women's bodies and minds through traditional Chinese wisdom / Xiaolan Zhao ; with Kanae Kinoshita.

Includes index.

ISBN: 978-0-679-31419-6

          1. Women—Health and hygiene. 2. Medicine, Chinese. 3. Alternative medicine. I. Kinoshita, Kanae II. Title.

RA778.Z53 2007   613'.04244   C2006-902108-2

Image Credits

p. 11 Studying the Yin Yang Symbol, hanging scroll (detail). © The Trustees of the British Museum.

pp. 19, 62, 96–98, 129–32, 156, 168, 188, 189, 208–10, 290–292 by Hu Yaxong.

p. 103 Lotus and Ducks, late thirteenth-century Chinese painting on silk, unsigned (detail). Reproduced by permission of the Saint Louis Art Museum. Funds given by an anonymous donor, the Ruth Peters MacCarthy Charitable Trust, Dr. Patricia L. O'Neal, Dr. and Mrs. Andrew Luh, Mr. and Mrs. Robert E. Kresko, and an anonymous donor.

p. 137 Amorous couple, ink on silk, by Jiao Bingzhen (1622–1723 AD). Courtesy of Lina Shen.

Text Permissions

Every effort has been made to contact copyright holders; in the event of an inadvertent omission or error, please notify the publisher.

Eliot, T.S., "East Coker," *Four Quartets*, Copyright © 1944 T.S. Eliot, Faber and Faber Limited.

Maciocia, Giovanni, *Obstetrics and Gynecology in Chinese Medicine*, Copyright © 1998 Giovanni Maciocia, Churchill Livingstone.

Cover and text design: Kelly Hill

Printed and bound in the United States of America

10 9 8 7 6 5 4 3 2 1

To my grandmother,
who taught me so much

Contents

PART FOUR

Clouds and Rain

PART FIVE

Ripening the Fruit

PART SIX

Golden Month

PART SEVEN

Second Spring

Foreword

When I first entered Xiaolan Zhao's clinic many years ago, I experienced a beautiful healing space where I was surrounded by care and compassion. Xiaolan gave me acupuncture and massage, and it was a wonderfully healing treatment. Since then, many of my friends, family and patients have passed through her office—in fact, she is the only doctor my husband would ever go to.

Xiaolan's new book, *Reflections of the Moon on Water*, is a labour of love that brings the healing atmosphere of her practice to the world. This enlightening and invaluable book should be at the bedside of every woman. It is a compelling look at the stages of a woman's life and includes a wealth of practical suggestions for living them in harmony with nature's rhythms to maintain health and prevent disease.

In Western medicine, we have medicalized the natural and healthy stages of a woman's life. We over-prescribe birth control pills, hormonal medications, tranquilizers, antidepressants, and many other medications, much to the detriment of women's health. In contrast, in Chinese medicine, the stages of a woman's life are honoured and celebrated. Menstruation is referred to as Heavenly Water, pregnancy is called Ripening the Fruit, postpartum is known as Golden Month, and menopause is called Second Spring. Golden Month, the prescribed period of rest following childbirth, is one of my favourite concepts in Chinese medicine. During Golden Month, the mother and babe are encircled in a cocoon of love and nurturing by their family, completely cared for day and night so that the energy depleted during childbirth can be replenished. I think there would be far less postpartum depression and sheer hardship for women in the West if at least some of these principles were adhered to.

The ancient traditions of Chinese medicine are needed more than ever in our society where women are increasingly pressured to be superwomen and are fatigued, stressed and sleep-deprived beyond endurance. And breast cancer and heart disease, autoimmune diseases in which the body attacks its own tissues, are all on the increase.

In the Chinese art of feng shui, we make our environment harmonious for the flow of Qi, or life force. Our most valuable possession, our body, the house we live in, must be put in similar balance in order to optimize our health and ensure a healthy and vibrant Second Spring. This book will enable you to care for and thoroughly enjoy the body that you're in.

Carolyn DeMarco, MD
Author of *Take Charge of Your Body: Women's Health Advisor*

Introduction

In 1986, I was working as a general surgeon in the emergency department of the biggest hospital in the city of Kunming, China, when a twenty-four-year-old woman named Jiayu was rushed in. She was vomiting bright red blood, and from its colour I assumed it was coming from a hemorrhage in her upper digestive tract. I, together with my medical team, operated immediately, but could not find the source of the bleeding. Three hours later, Jiayu was again throwing up blood.

Mystified and concerned, we consulted the chairman, the head doctor of the hospital. He thought we should again do exploratory surgery but this time to look farther down for the hemorrhage, to the small intestine, pancreas and gallbladder. An hour or two into the operation, using all the medical technology at our disposal, we still could not locate the source of Jiayu's bleeding. Everyone was shocked. We'd successfully performed countless abdominal surgeries to treat acute conditions, but this time we were at a loss. Within a matter of hours, Jiayu was again vomiting blood.

We decided to call an emergency meeting with the hospital's top surgeons. All five were at home sleeping in their beds when the nurse called them, since it was the middle of the night. But they soon arrived at the hospital and quickly changed into their surgical clothes. Together we operated for the third time, carefully looking everywhere we'd already looked. But there was no wound, no internal bleeding—everything looked clean. Approximately twenty-four hours had passed since Jiayu had been admitted, and we were no closer to understanding why she was vomiting blood. We felt helpless.

Jiayu's family had remained at the hospital the entire time, and to this day, I can still remember her husband, who was understandably distraught, unable to stand up or articulate a thought. All he could do was sob out his love for his wife. Hope was fading for him and their beautiful eight-month-old daughter. The chairman of the hospital looked at me and said, "Xiaolan, do whatever you think may help. She's almost gone." He knew that I was also a doctor of Traditional Chinese Medicine (TCM) and was asking me to use anything from that knowledge to save Jiayu.

I had studied several traditional Chinese herbal formulas that were supposed to be effective in stopping hemorrhaging. One in particular, called the Yellow Earth Formula, came to mind. I went to my office and looked up the formula in a reference book. I gave Jiayu's family the list of ingredients and instructions. They would have to prepare the remedy at home and bring it to the hospital, since we had no facilities for cooking herbs. Within four hours they returned with the herbal remedy.

By now, Jiayu had lost so much blood she was unconscious and extremely weak. She was alive only because of the intravenous fluids and blood transfusions we had given her. We administered the herbs through a tube in her nose and waited. Two hours passed and she did not vomit. Three hours passed, then six hours, then twelve turned into twenty-four. Something in the herbal formula had stopped the bleeding.

For me, this experience was an incredibly powerful demonstration of the effectiveness of TCM. Previously, I had witnessed herbs releasing symptoms of a cold, or acupuncture relieving sinus problems, or *Tui Na* (Chinese massage) alleviating back pain. But I'd never witnessed Chinese medicine saving someone's life in an emergency situation in which Western medicine had failed. I had been educated in medical school, in the rational world of evidence-based science. I based my thinking on one plus one equals two, and believed that problems had solutions that could be logically figured out. But the effectiveness of the Yellow Earth formula could not be explained by Western medicine. On top of this, the cause of Jiayu's bleeding remained a mystery. We never found the source of the hemorrhaging.

Biases come into play when we seek to understand TCM through the eyes of Western medicine. The development of TCM began more than 5,000 years ago, 4,500 years before the scientific traditions of the West, in a culture with a unique view of the world and that forbade human dissection. Ancient practitioners had to rely on their powers of observation and trial and error to develop a medical system and terminology. As a result, they had a different understanding of the body and disease than we do in the West. But after centuries of assessment and evaluation, TCM has withstood the test of time. It is still an integral part of the health-care system in China and is practised alongside Western medicine in many hospitals. Indeed, doctors of Western medicine and of TCM receive the same amount of education and training and are equally respected. People seek out either Western or Chinese medicine, depending on the nature of their illness. For acute problems such as heart attacks, they'll go to a hospital emergency department for Western-style health care. For chronic conditions, such as arthritis or migraine headaches, they will usually consult a TCM practitioner. Each discipline has its own particular strengths, so combining the two can work very well. Doctors of Western medicine will often invite a TCM practitioner to consult on a particular case, and vice versa.

In the West, TCM is still considered an alternative medicine. In recent decades, however, hundreds of studies have been undertaken in an effort to give TCM a firmer scientific basis. For instance, a series of controlled studies of acupuncture has revealed its efficacy in the treatment of various conditions, including headaches, lower back pain, carpal tunnel syndrome, stroke, addiction, infertility and mitigating the side effects from cancer treatment. In 2004, the results of a landmark study funded by the National Institutes of Health (NIH) found that patients with osteoarthritis in their knees showed a 40 per cent decrease in pain, and a 40 per cent improvement in function when treated with acupuncture.

Western science has proven that acupuncture works, but it still cannot explain *how* it works. It doesn't accept the seemingly irrational TCM explanation, which holds that acupuncture needles inserted into specific points along our Meridian pathways can unblock the flow of *Qi,* or vital energy, which affects our health. Sometimes phenomena are inexplicable but nonetheless powerful in their capacity to affect us.

In 1992, I came to Canada and set up a TCM clinic in Toronto, where I now treat more than 7,000 patients who experience benefits through Chinese medicine. In general they have difficulty explaining the relief or well-being they feel. They may not be able to apply logic to what has taken place in their bodies, but they begin to trust that the practices of Chinese medicine can help them.

Many of my female patients come to me with similar health problems. My heart goes out to them. I see women struggling with fatigue, depression, menstrual difficulties, infertility, chronic pain and cancer—especially breast cancer. I give them treatments that combine acupuncture, Tui Na and Chinese herbs, and as they begin to experience effective results, most want to learn more about Chinese medicine. I decided that a book like *Reflections of the Moon on Water,* which would focus on women's health and make Chinese medicine accessible to any reader, could be helpful.

To many Westerners, Chinese medicine sounds complicated and esoteric. They find discussions of Yin and Yang, or the life energy known as Qi, intimidating. In fact, Chinese medicine is very straightforward and easy to understand and apply. It draws on nature, ancient knowledge of herbs and the body's own healing resources. Sometimes, I might treat a patient's sinus condition with eucalyptus or other familiar herbs, and she'll say, "Oh, that smells just like what my grandmother used to give me." So much of Chinese medicine is based on intuition and common sense.

I knew that Chinese medicine could treat illness, but one of the areas I wanted to focus on in this book was the prevention of disease. Historically, Chinese medical practitioners only received payment if their patients stayed healthy. After all, if patients became ill, they wouldn't be able to work to earn the money they'd need to pay the doctor. Clearly, it was in everyone's interest to prevent people from getting sick.

This preventive approach stresses harmony and balance in our daily lives by paying attention to what we eat, how we exercise, and the way we handle our emotions, our sexual lives, work and sleep. It is the balance we maintain among these different aspects that creates more energy and protects us from getting sick. TCM asks us to take responsibility for our health, and supports us in this process. This is what I find so valuable about this approach to health: TCM is not just about treating illness, it's about living life with more balance, self-awareness and vitality.

Many women have a hard time trusting their bodies and connecting to the positive aspects of the female cycle. No matter what country we live in, our experiences in male-oriented societies are similar: There is a lack of cultural support for women as we move through some of the important transitions. As a result, we have a hard time trusting our bodies and connecting to the positive aspects of the female cycle. In the West, we often view menstruation as a nuisance or a pain ("the curse") rather than as an opportunity to develop a new relationship with our bodies. We may see childbirth as an interruption in our lives rather than something that creates a new feeling of connectedness. We gloomily think of menopause as the end of youth, rather than as the beginning of a time of spiritual growth and new-found freedoms. Female sexuality in the West is often associated with youthfulness and body image. We're all supposed to be a size two until we're old, and then that's the end of sex for us. Chinese medicine, on the other hand, understands sexuality as a lifelong, vital aspect of health and longevity. Sexual energy is just one current of the energy that flows through us and keeps us strong.

At my clinic, patients often open up to me and talk about what's bothering them emotionally. As acupuncture releases the flow of energy in the body, feelings frequently surface. In TCM, the mind and body are inseparable, and chronic physical symptoms are often linked to unresolved emotions. I'm struck by the fears and anxieties that women experience in relation to their bodies, their sexual lives, illness and the prospect of getting old. These fears drain their health and depress them. According to TCM, these negative feelings contribute to the development of disease.

How can we take care of our health if we don't cultivate a basic level of love and respect for our bodies, and for the different seasons of a woman's life? In writing this book, I hope to encourage women to develop a kinder, more compassionate relationship with themselves. We can become aware of new ways to relate to our bodies, hearts and minds, and this kind of empowerment is an important part of my practice, where I ask questions such as: How can we reconnect to our true nature? How can we convince ourselves that our bodily rhythms are natural and good?

I am passionate about sharing the gifts of Traditional Chinese Medicine and want to show women how they can use it to prevent illness, protect their vitality and gain awareness of their own capacity to stay well and heal themselves. TCM takes a collaborative approach to health, asking us to connect with nature. It assumes that the capacity to heal lies inside us, not just in the hands of medical experts. Western medicine sometimes pathologizes the natural transitions of a woman's life. We talk more about the risk of postpartum depression than about the deepening of emotion that accompanies new motherhood. At menopause, we talk more about the need for hormone replacement or other medications, rather than the opportunity for spiritual exploration and evolution that comes with age. TCM treats the phases of a woman's life as healthy transitions and offers ways to support us as we move through them.

In TCM, disease is an expression of the whole person— body, mind and spirit—in relation to the environment. Chinese medicine doesn't just treat isolated symptoms in iso-lated body parts. It gently encourages an awareness of the self as a whole, which in turn promotes strength and healing. As a result, I've tried to organize this book using the same holistic principles, instead of dividing it into discussions of separate body parts and medical conditions. I begin the book with a brief introduction to the basic principles of TCM— the concept of Yin and Yang, Qi, the Zang-Fu Organs and the Five Phases. To distinguish between what Western medicine means by certain organs and fluids and the TCM versions, I've capitalized the references to the Chinese organs and flu-ids. Please bear with me here—these concepts may be new to you and difficult perhaps to take in, but having some knowl-edge of them is necessary to understand Chinese medicine. Don't worry if you don't grasp it all at once; the concepts will become clearer as you read the following chapters, and you can always return to Part 1 for reference. Elsewhere in the book, I've tried to keep my theoretical explanations rooted in stories drawn from my own life and the experiences of my patients.

The book follows the natural narrative of a woman's life as it evolves from puberty, through pregnancy and childbirth, towards menopause and onwards. I've used traditional Chinese terms for these, which are poetic and nature-based. So, Part Two, on menstruation, is called "Heavenly Water," and Part Five, on pregnancy, is entitled "Ripening the Fruit." The time after childbirth is known as "Golden Month" (Part Six). Menopause (Part Seven) is referred to as "Second Spring." I've also included a section, called "Lotus Blossoms" (Part Three), devoted to breast health, which is so problematic in the West—one in nine women will experience breast cancer—and so intimately connected with each stage of the female cycles. Part Four, "Clouds and Rain," is about sexuality, and explores how we can deepen and direct our sexual energies throughout life. I hope that this framework will help give readers a sense of the uniquely integrated approach of TCM.

The title, *Reflections of the Moon on Water*, evokes the archetypal aspects of the feminine that we each embody. In TCM, both the moon and water have been symbolically connected with Yin, the feminine, and many cultures compare women's evolution from young woman to mother to matriarch with the transformation of the moon in her phases. The title is also meant to suggest the transformational possibilities that arise when we share ourselves with others. Just as I have shared my knowledge and experience of Chinese medicine with my patients, the wonderful women I've met in Canada have shown themselves to me, and in so doing have illuminated parts of myself that were previously hidden—like the dark side of the moon. The luminous light of our wholeness is reflected in each of us, for all of us to see. It is my hope that by sharing my understanding and experience of Traditional Chinese Medicine and offering stories from my life and the lives of my wise and courageous patients, you will be equipped with knowledge and practices to help you in your transitions. Also, it is my heartfelt wish that this book can help us reconnect to what is authentic within us, in a healing journey towards wholeness.

Part One

ORCHIDS UNFOLDING IN
THE UNIVERSE

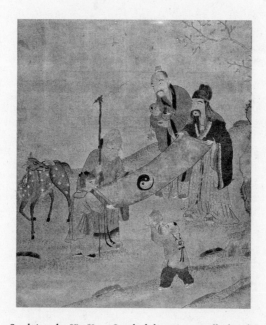

Studying the Yin Yang Symbol, hanging scroll (detail)

CHAPTER ONE

As Above, So Below

When a practitioner of Western medicine is asked about the human body, she might describe it "as an organism that can be separated into components. It is like a machine, in that the different organs and systems in the body can be further taken apart, examined and understood." As a practitioner of Traditional Chinese Medicine, however, I would say, "There is a whole person, including the body, a unified whole. All aspects of an individual—physical, emotional, mental and spiritual—are interconnected and interdependent, and any one part cannot be understood except in relation to the whole. Each of us is a unified organic body-mind-spirit." When a patient comes into my office, I observe her expression, the luminosity of her eyes, her complexion, her demeanour, the build of her body, her posture and the way she smells. I take her pulse and examine her tongue. I ask questions to open a dialogue, and listen carefully to what she says. I use all of my senses to find the outward signs and symptoms that reflect the dynamic of what is going on in her body, and this method of diagnosis has been passed down to me from ancient Chinese practitioners. The way they understood and described the workings of the human body was based on their analysis and shaped by Taoist philosophy, which held that humans are an aspect of nature and, as such, are governed by the same natural laws as the universe. Therefore, they reasoned, each individual is a miniature universe, or microcosm, with analogies to the larger universe. The ancient Chinese medical treatise *Huang Di Nei Jing,* or *The Yellow Emperor's Classic of Internal Medicine,* explains: "Heaven has the sun and moon, humans have two eyes . . . Heaven has thunder and lightning, humans have sound and speech; Heaven has wind and rain, humans have joy and anger. . . . Heaven has winter and summer, humans have hot and cold. . . . Heaven has morning and evening, humans go to sleep and awake."

The Taoists saw the universe as organized and harmonious. They believed that if we lived according to the laws of the universe we, too, would be harmonious. One way to do this would be to act in harmony with the seasons, by going to bed when the sun goes down, waking up when the sun comes up, dressing appropriately for the weather and eating foods that are in season where we live. The changes in behaviour should mirror the changes occurring on a universal level, because what is beneficial for the macrocosm (the whole of nature) is beneficial for the individual (the microcosm), and vice versa.

This concept, seen from another perspective, would view what is supportive of the environment as supportive of living organisms. For example, rain sustains trees and plants and fills the lakes, rivers and streams, which provide us with drinking water. On a microcosmic level, water is needed by every part of my body. Consequently, it is not possible to isolate one part of my body or one symptom without due consideration of the rest of my body. We would also not treat one condition without understanding the impact on the rest of the body, or what may have caused the specific symptom. If someone came into my office with a red, itchy rash, I would not only look at her skin but would also ask about her gastrointestinal health and her breathing, since all three are associated in TCM. I would also be interested to know whether she'd recently experienced any significant loss in her life, since sadness can be a factor in Lung disorders, which in turn can lead to an inflammation of the skin.

All disorders and disease are the result of an imbalance in the body. The ancient Chinese perceived everything in the universe, including us, as an interplay between two opposing forces that are constantly shifting: cold in winter changes into heat in summer; dark of night gives way to daylight; rest is replaced by activity. These two opposing forces are known as Yin and Yang.

YIN AND YANG

All things in nature, as well as all activities in life, have two opposing aspects: a Yin aspect and a Yang aspect. *Yin* means "the shadowy side of the mountain," while *Yang* translates as "the sunny side of the mountain." Yin is associated with shade, cold, contraction, the moon, water, inactivity, the feminine and matter. Yang is regarded as brightness, hot, expansion, the sun, fire, activity, the masculine and energy. These apparently opposing aspects are two sides of the same coin.

Hot and cold are characteristics of temperature; day and night are aspects of time. They exist only in relation to each other, for how could there be night without day, or a back without a front?

The dynamic tension and constant transformation that takes place between Yin and Yang is what creates the energy that nourishes nature, and human life. Yin and Yang are like the pull between positive and negative electrical forces, or the simple truism that "opposites attract." Yin is female and Yang is male. And of course it is the union of these two kinds of energy that creates new life. Yin and Yang make the world go round.

The symbol of Yin and Yang is a circle, half-dark (Yin), half-light (Yang), divided by a curving line, which represents the ceaseless movement and dynamic that underlies all life, as well as the harmonious balance that exists between opposing forces (see Figure 1). There is a dark dot in the light half, and a light dot in the dark half, illustrating that phenomena are never exclusively Yin or Yang. For example, I am short relative to a six-foot person, but I am tall compared to a four-foot child. The dots also show that the source of their opposite state is inherent within all phenomena. For example, as soon as we are born, we have the possibility to die. This concept of Yin and Yang reflects the Eastern view that opposites do not have to compete, conquer or come into conflict, since each aspect contains, complements and balances the other.

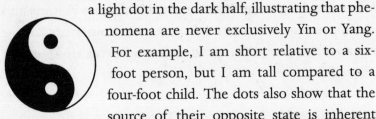

Figure 1: Yin Yang

Like everything in the universe, we are a combination of Yin and Yang. Our heads, because they are above, are Yang, while our feet are Yin. Our backs are Yang and our fronts are Yin. TCM describes every part of our bodies, including our organs and fluids, as predominantly Yin or Yang and sees health as the capacity to maintain a balance between the two within ourselves by living in harmony with the natural principles of the universe. If Yin or Yang are out of balance, illness may result. If we have an excess of Yin, we have a deficiency in Yang, and our symptoms might include cold hands and feet, slow pulse and tiredness. We may find we prefer yoga to aerobics, may need time to make decisions and tend to be good listeners. We may speak softly or quietly. If we have an excess of Yang, we have a deficiency in Yin, and our symptoms might include constipation, dry lips and excessive sweating. We might find we get warm easily, like to keep active and naturally initiate activity. We do not hesitate to go after what we want.

In China, the majority of my patients had a Yang Deficiency. In Canada, I have many patients with a Deficiency in Yin energy. I think this is a reflection of the overriding quality of Yang in Canadian society, and in the Western world in general. Activity, movement, speed, growth, expansion, youth and patriarchy epitomize our culture. Western society is not all Yang, but its excess is apparent in the imbalances found in my Canadian patients. To balance the Yang quality of Western culture, I suggest Yin activity, such as inward moments of stillness. Walking among trees, reflecting on the sunset, sitting quietly or meditating on a rock all embody Yin characteristics. These activities possess qualities of quiescence versus qualities of activity.

You may be wondering what gives rise to these excesses or deficiencies. It is the dynamic movement of *Qi* (pronounced "chee"), a concept fundamental to Chinese medicine.

UNDERSTANDING QI

In the Western world there is no equivalent word for Qi, though it is often described as "vital energy." This definition, however, does not entirely capture its meaning. Qi is the natural enlivening energy of the universe that activates change and movement. It is the creative force that permeates everything: the twinkling stars, a babbling brook and a decomposing organism are all found within the cause-and-effect power of Qi. It is like the wind in its ability to affect change and drive activity.

Qi is the energy that creates life, our vitality, the vital force that underlies our bodies, minds, hearts and spirits. It is immaterial and invisible, and yet has the capability to produce material and visible effects, as when through conception, a baby is formed. Qi is also transformative in character. For example, it gives rise to the materiality of our bodies, just as water can change into ice. As ice thaws and melts, it transforms back to water. Similarly, we may feel that when we die we become spirit. The two Chinese characters that form the ideogram for

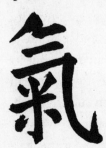

Figure 2: Qi

Qi (see Figure 2) mean "vapour" or "steam," and "uncooked rice" or "grain." The steam that rises from cooking rice represents Qi in a formless state, while the rice symbolizes the substantial and material aspect of matter. Inherent in the Chinese word is the transformative and changing Essence of Qi from the material to the immaterial and back again.

The movement of Qi in our bodies affects all our activities. As a child in China, I was taught, "When Qi gathers, so the physical body is formed; when it disperses, so the body dies." Qi is the energy that stimulates activity—our capacity to digest our food, move our legs, think. This energy can also manifest as resentment or the lump in our throats when we are sad. Qi is a radically different way for those of us in the West to view ourselves. But we do have phrases such as "full of life" to describe people who are energetic and alive. On some profound level we have a sense that there is a connection between the movement of a vital energetic force and life.

Western science has not proven the existence of Qi—it cannot be seen with a microscope, or dissected or CAT-scanned. However, this doesn't mean that we can't *feel* Qi. Here is a simple exercise you can try: Bring your hands in front of your belly, palms facing each other. Slowly bring your hands close to each other without letting them touch. Now move them away from each other. Repeat this action slowly (see Figure 3). Note the mild tension, warmth, tingling, pulsation or pressure between

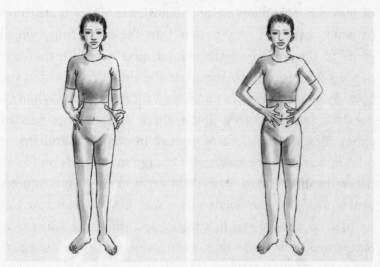

Figure 3: Exercise to Feel Qi

your palms. The air may feel denser in the space between your hands. This is Qi. Don't try to comprehend Qi with your rational mind. Try to feel it.

As you move your palms near each other, slowly and gently extend your fingers and flex your palms (see Figure 3). As you move them apart, let your hands relax. Now gently move the fingers of your right hand over your left palm. Without touching it, stroke your left palm with the tips of your fingers. There may be a tingling sensation. This is Qi coming out of your fingers.

Though Western science does not recognize Qi, Chinese practitioners have been working with harmonizing its flow for more than 3,000 years. Qi moves through the body through a network of pathways, or Meridians. One of the hardest aspects of Chinese medicine for Westerners to grasp is the concept of Meridians, which are the invisible channels that flow over the length of the body and connect the vital organs to other parts of the body. Meridians are not identified in Western anatomy. In acupuncture, however, it is into these conduits, which come to the surface of the skin at specific points, that tiny needles are inserted to stimulate the flow of Qi within the body. When Qi flows harmoniously, there is health. When Qi does not flow smoothly, illness arises. Acupuncture needles either increase the flow of energy in certain Meridians or calm it, restoring the balance of energy in the body and facilitating health. This is how TCM explains the way acupuncture works. Western doctors have seen how acupuncture can be used as anaesthesia in surgery and think the effect may have something to do with stimulating nerves to distribute natural painkillers. We may not have a rational explanation for how or why acupuncture works, but its effectiveness cannot be doubted.

Qi is essential for our bodies to produce Blood. Qi is also what circulates Blood through our blood vessels and Meridians. The relationship between Blood and Qi is interdependent: Inasmuch as Qi is needed for the production and movement of Blood, Blood feeds our Organs that create and support Qi. So Qi and Blood are inseparable. Without the movement of Blood, there would be no vehicle to transport the energetic, formless Qi. Conversely, Qi provides the motive force that animates Blood. Obviously, TCM's concept of Blood is different than that of the West. Blood refers not only to the fluid that moves through our blood vessels, but also to the energetic quality that activates Blood to nourish and circulate through our body. Since Blood is Yin and Qi is Yang, harmony between the two symbolizes a unitary whole that is represented by health.

Blood is stored in our Liver and Qi is stored in our Kidneys. I tell my patients, "Chinese medicine doctors are very familiar with the major organs of Western medicine's anatomy. But although they may have similar names, they are very different." Chinese medicine views the organs as physical-anatomical structures, with similar functions as in Western medicine, but with a broader energetic sphere of functioning and influence that includes the Meridians that connect the organs to other parts of the body. These paired Organ networks, or systems, are referred to as the Zang-Fu Organs.

THE ZANG-FU ORGANS

The term *Zang-Fu* itself is used to describe the principle of Yin and Yang as applied to the Organs. Yin Organs are referred to as Zang, and Yang Organs are referred to as Fu. Each of the five Zang Organs—the Liver, Heart, Spleen, Lung and Kidneys—have corresponding Fu Organs—the Gallbladder, Small Intestine, Stomach, Large Intestine and Urinary Bladder respectively. Each of the Organ pairs is associated with a sense organ, such as the eyes and ears, and also tissues (see Table 1). The Liver is responsible for the smooth movement of Qi and Blood, the storage of Blood, the governing of tendons and the nourishment of the eyes. (This might sound odd to you until you remember that liver diseases like hepatitis cause the whites of the eyes to yellow.)

The Zang-Fu Organ theory describes our bodies and our Organs' functions in terms of interdependence with all the other Organ systems. The Spleen transforms the food we eat into food Qi that is needed by the Heart to make Blood. The Kidneys provide Qi to the Heart to manufacture Blood. The Lungs help to transport food Qi to the Heart to support Blood production. The Blood circulates through the vessels in our body as a result of the Qi of our Heart. The proper functioning of our Spleen helps to ensure that Blood stays within the vessel walls. The Liver both governs the smooth movement of Qi and stores blood and controls its volume. Thus, each of the Organ systems maintains a close relationship with the others, and our health depends on their harmonious workings. How well they function is a result of how smoothly our Qi and Blood move through these systems. If the flow becomes blocked in any one Organ, there is a "Stagnation" in that

Organ. If there isn't enough Qi, there is a "Deficiency." If there is too much Qi, there is an "Excess" in that Organ. And because each of the Organ systems maintains a close relationship with the others, these imbalances have a profound effect on all the other Organs, and ultimately may lead to disease.

Thousands of years of observation and clinical practice have allowed Chinese medicine to describe the symptomatic

TABLE 1: THE ZANG-FU ORGANS

ZANG ORGAN	The Liver	The Heart	The Spleen	The Lung	The Kidneys
PRIMARY FUNCTION	Stores Blood, governs free movement of Qi	Governs transformations of Qi from food into Blood, responsible for thinking, conciousness and Spirit (*Shen*)	Governs the transformation and transportation of food into Qi, holds Blood within the vessels	Governs respiration, transformation of Qi from air, forwards the Qi transformed from food to the Heart	Stores Qi, governs reproduction, development and growth
FU ORGAN	Gallbladder Governs storage and secretion of bile	Small Intestine Receives digested food and separates "clean" from "turbid"	Stomach Transforms food and liquids	Large Intestine Responsible for the elimination of feces	Urinary Bladder Responsible for the storage and excretion of urine
SENSE ORGAN	Eyes	Tongue	Mouth	Nose	Ears
TISSUE	Tendon, Ligaments, Nails	Blood Vessels	Muscle, Fat	Skin, Hair	Bone, Marrow, Brain

expression of deep Organ or Meridian imbalances. For example, Stagnating Liver Qi may be expressed as migraine headaches and irregular periods. Together, the symptoms form a pattern that points to the underlying imbalance that is causing the problems. The relationships between the Organs can be explained by the classifications and laws of movement provided by the Five Phases theory. It describes how Qi interacts and what is needed to bring it into harmony.

THE FIVE PHASES THEORY

The harmonious movement of Qi in the world is a reflection of the balance of five basic phases: Wood, Fire, Earth, Metal and Water. Wood promotes Fire; Fire burns Wood, thereby promoting Earth; within Earth there is Metal; and Metal, melted by Fire, promotes Water (see Figure 4). All phenomena in the natural world correspond to one of the Five Phases, which are constantly moving and changing. For example, Spring corresponds to Wood, Summer to Fire, Late Summer to Earth, Fall to Metal and Winter to Water. The Phases aren't attributes that were arbitrarily assigned to things by the ancient Chinese. Instead, the qualities of each phase describe the characteristics, forms and functions of the phenomenon it is assigned to. For example, Wood represents active phases and growth, which is the reason that it is associated with Spring. The seasons change the way the Phases transform. Spring leads to Summer, which leads to Late Summer, then Fall and Winter.

In addition to the seasons, the Five Phases are used to describe aspects of climate, colour, flavours—virtually everything in the universe. And because each of us is a microcosm, we each possess within us a unique combination of the influ-

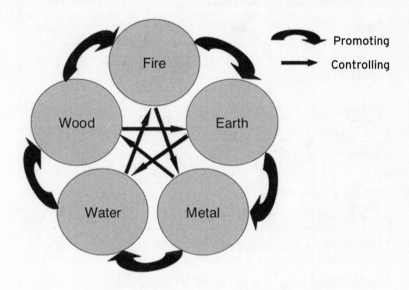

Figure 4: The Relationships Between the Five Phases

ences of the Five Phases. Each of our five major Organs corresponds with one of the Phases. Table 2 illustrates how the human body is related to the Five Phases, life cycles, emotions, flavours, tendencies, virtues, seasons, climates, directions and colours.

Because the Heart has warming properties, it is associated with Fire. The Liver is associated with Wood, the Spleen with Earth, the Lungs with Metal, and the Kidneys with Water. These classifications help explain how the Organs function in relation to each other. The theory also tells us what happens when there is disharmony, and Chinese practitioners use it to diagnose and treat Organ imbalances. For example, if a woman is experiencing hot flashes, this is a symptom that her Fire element is too strong. Fire that is burning out of control

TABLE 2: THE FIVE PHASES AND THEIR ASSOCIATIONS

PHASE	Wood	Fire	Earth	Metal	Water
ZANG ORGAN	Liver	Heart	Spleen	Lung	Kidney
LIFE-CYCLE PHASE	Infancy	Youth	Adult	Old Age	Death
EMOTION	Anger	Joy	Over-thinking	Grief	Fear, Anxiety
FLAVOUR	Sour	Bitter	Sweet	Pungent	Bitter
TENDENCY	Assertiveness	Expression	Cooperation	Discrimination	Contemplation
VIRTUE	Generosity	Gratitude	Faith	Compassion	Wisdom
SEASON	Spring	Summer	Late Summer	Autumn	Winter
CLIMATE	Windy	Hot	Damp	Dry	Cold
DIRECTION	East	South	Centre	West	North
COLOUR	Green	Red	Yellow	White	Black

indicates that the Wood element is too dry. It is not being sufficiently nourished by Water. Water is needed to control body temperature and moisten eyes, sexual organs, joints and muscles. Since the Kidneys are associated with Water, hot flashes are a symptom of Deficient Kidney Qi, specifically Kidney Yin. Other symptoms of this deficiency would be insomnia, vaginal dryness and sore joints and muscles. Treating this condition would entail strengthening Kidney Qi, specifically Yin, or nourishing the body's Water to control the Fire, through acupuncture, Tui Na and herbs that are a bit salty (a flavour associated with the Kidneys).

In this way, Chinese medicine is all about restoring harmony in the body. Rather than pinpointing disease-causing bacteria and using antibiotics to fight them off, TCM locates the weakness or imbalance that is causing susceptibility to illness, and then helps the person achieve a harmonious and balanced state of well-being through supportive herbs, acupuncture, Tui Na and lifestyle recommendations. Health is not just the absence of symptoms; it is the harmonious and balanced functioning of the body. Many variables contribute to this balance, such as heredity, lifestyle, the environment we live in and how we respond to and are impacted by it. The next chapter examines, in depth, what is needed to maintain balance.

CHAPTER TWO

Maintaining Harmony

Moving towards well-being depends on the harmonious functioning of our physical, emotional and spiritual aspects—the three levels of energy known as the "Three Treasures." They are *Jing*, or "Essence," *Qi*, the natural enlivening energy of the universe, and *Shen*, meaning "Spirit" or "Mind." Jing is inherited from our parents and is the most substantive and material of the Three Treasures. It is closely related to our genetic blueprint and is the substance our bodies are made of. Qi is what enlivens us and gives rise to our emotions. Shen, or Spirit, the most subtle energy of the Three Treasures, depends on the vitality of Qi and Jing for its strength and vigour. When the body is healthy and strong, and the emotions are sound, free flowing and appropriately expressed, our spiritual health can deepen.

All Three Treasures are intimately interwoven and must be consciously cultivated and balanced to maintain optimal health. Looking after ourselves from the perspective of the

Three Treasures requires that we become aware of, and bring into harmony, our emotional states, lifestyle, diet and our interaction with our environment to cultivate spiritual wholeness. Striving to bring into balance the different aspects of our being, as represented in the Three Treasures, is the ultimate objective of Chinese medicine. We are encouraged to take this responsibility, as this forms the first barrier of defence against invading disease and is considered the highest form of medicine—prevention.

The preventative approach focuses on maintaining and vitalizing the strength of our Three Treasures by avoiding unfavourable circumstances. When harmony with nature is upset, when moderation gives rise to excess, ill health and disease will manifest. There is great emphasis in Chinese medicine on conducting our lives in ways that nurture and enhance the Three Treasures, so as not to deplete these essential energies. By making proper choices in what we eat, how we exercise, how we deal with our emotions and when we work and rest, it is not beyond anyone to help prevent disease and promote personal health. In fact, no amount of treatment by a practitioner will overcome an unhealthy diet or a poor lifestyle.

In Traditional Chinese Medicine, there are three categories of causes of disharmony: Exterior Causes, Interior Causes and Neither Exterior nor Interior Causes (see Table 3). These pathogenic, or disease-causing, factors can disturb the balance of the Three Treasures within our body and produce a hospitable environment for disease.

EXTERIOR CAUSES OF DISHARMONY

The Exterior Causes, also known as the "Six Excesses," are Cold, Wind, Heat, Dampness, Dryness and Fire. Because these pathogenic factors are related to climate, we must take care to dress appropriately for the weather. Sometimes we dress according to the calendar rather than current weather conditions. We know it is June, so we dress lightly, perhaps ignoring that it is an unusually chilly June. Or in winter, we bundle up because it is January, not paying attention to the fact that it is an inordinately mild winter. We should also be aware of Dry and Damp conditions, taking care to drink sufficient liquids, and to cover our heads and feet when it is raining. Dampness, like Cold, can lodge in our Meridians or impede the flow of Qi in the Organs. In the summer, I often have patients come to see me with stiff, painful necks. This is more often than not caused by the air conditioners in their offices blowing cold air at them all day. I give them acupuncture and Tui Na treatments and advise them to wear scarves at work.

If a child in China develops a severe cold, her mother does not ask where she might have picked up the virus, but whether her child was wearing her heavy jacket yesterday when she was out playing, or if she was warm when she went to sleep the previous night. It is the quantity and quality of our Qi that determines whether Exterior factors will upset it and we will fall ill to a cold, while others similarly exposed do not. There is a well-known Chinese saying: "If good Qi is inside your body, no evil can catch you."

INTERIOR CAUSES OF DISHARMONY

The Interior Causes of disharmony are our seven emotions: joy, anger, anxiety, obsession, sadness, horror and fear. If we experience any of these emotions excessively over a sustained period of time, our flow of energy will be adversely affected and we may become ill. Does this mean that we are to feel only in moderation? No, we are human and we are always feeling deeply. What is important is that there is a balance in our emotions. Over the course of a week, for example, we may feel great joy, anger, anxiety, sadness and fear, and there may be

TABLE 3: EXTERIOR, INTERIOR AND NEITHER EXTERIOR NOR INTERIOR CAUSES OF DISEASE

EXTERIOR CAUSES	**Six Excesses** • Cold • Dampness • Wind • Dryness • Heat or Fire • Summer heat
INTERIOR CAUSES	**Seven Emotions** • Joy • Sadness • Anger • Horror • Anxiety • Fear • Obsession, over-pensiveness

NEITHER EXTERIOR NOR INTERIOR CAUSES	• Too much or too little physical exertion
	• Lack of sexual activity, and frequent
	  pregnancies
	• Diet
	  • Moderation in and timing of consumption
	  • Nutritious foods
	• Constitution
	• Trauma

times when we do not experience these emotions strongly. If, however, over the course of the week we feel only anger or another emotion, our health may be compromised.

Chinese medicine has always acknowledged the connection between the body and mind, though Western science has only recently recognized it. Studies now show that stressful life events, such as the death of a spouse or loss of employment, greatly increase the risk of falling ill. Researchers have traced direct neurological pathways between the brain and the immune system. Many hospitals and medical centres now recommend programs of healing that include relaxation, meditation and visualization. This branch of medicine is known as psychoneuroimmunology.

In TCM, physical symptoms are not isolated from those of an emotional or mental nature. Conditions such as suicidal tendencies, psychosis and schizophrenia are all considered physical problems, arising from an energy imbalance in an Organ system.

The ancient Chinese believed that Qi was inherited from one's ancestors. Qi that gave rise to severe mental illness was considered faulty and reflected defects in one's ancestral lineage. Since Confucius placed strong emphasis on one's ancestors, these defects would have been cause for considerable guilt and shame. This may have been a contributing factor in the subsequent adoption by the Chinese of the view that psychological or mental symptoms were a result of the Causes of Disharmony, such as an unbalanced diet or one of the Six Excesses. Somatizing psychological illnesses in this way would have gone a long way in alleviating any shame arising from having them.

In TCM, the emotions are considered expressions of our Qi and accordingly will give rise to problems if they are blocked or inappropriately channelled or unexpressed. Encumbering the expression of our emotions includes denying them, or refusing to take notice and accept them. We inappropriately express our emotions when we cry instead of get angry in order to be "a good girl," or blame people for not listening when we should be confronting our failure to speak up. Sometimes these tactics keep us from dealing with emotions that are more threatening, such as our underlying fears.

The *Nei Jing* states: "It is known that all diseases arise from the upset of Qi: Anger pushes the Qi up, joy makes the Qi slacken, grief disperses the Qi, fear brings the Qi down, terror confuses the Qi, and anxiety causes the Qi to stagnate. Anger harms the Liver, joy the Heart, anxiety the Spleen, grief the Lungs and fear the Kidneys." Many Westerners are surprised to hear that joy, in particular, can have adverse effects on the body. But too much joy experienced continually over an extended length of time will put added stress on the Heart. Often the body will try to balance excessive happiness through tears.

Each of the Organ systems is connected with a specific emotion, and each of these emotions can affect a specific Organ system or, conversely, develop as a result of Organ imbalances. This means that if you have been grieving over a long period of time, and this sadness does not get transformed, it can energetically create disharmony in the flow of Lung Qi and physically manifest as a cold, asthma or even psoriasis. (Psoriasis is typically related to an imbalance in the Lungs, since skin is the tissue governed by the Lungs.) Also, if over a prolonged period of time, you have Deficient Lung Qi, you may find that you are prone to bouts of melancholy, or that tears flow at the slightest offence or sad story. If you worry or think too much, the Spleen Qi can become blocked, and you may experience digestive problems or bleed excessively during menstruation.

Consequently, the TCM practitioner diagnoses and treats emotional symptoms within the context of physical symptoms, searching for a pattern that addresses them all. For example, one of my patients was very introverted, had heavy, irregular periods, and suffered from temporomandibular jaw joint disease, a painful disorder of the jaw joints or the muscles that control the joints. All of these symptoms had clinical significance. They were interconnected manifestations of imbalances reflected in physical problems. The diagnosis was Liver Qi Stagnation, which contributed to her menstrual problems and the anger I detected smouldering under her quiet, unassuming facade. Her disease was also connected with Stomach Qi Excess, which may have developed from her Stagnating Liver Qi. Each of the symptoms was related to the other and could not be treated in isolation. Imbalances had occurred that were seriously affecting my patient on physical, emotional and mental levels. I gave her herbs, acupuncture, and Tui Na to smooth the flow of her Liver Qi, and her symptoms eventually dissipated.

The connection between the emotional, mental and physical is particularly significant in gynecological disorders, which involve many symptoms that are not physical in nature, such as the crying jags or angry outbursts that often precede a menstrual period. Every part of the mind-body is related and connected.

It is interesting to note that as much as there is a prevailing attitude in Chinese medicine that emotions are intimately related to a person's well-being, there is little talk *about* feelings. In fact, the understanding and expression of emotions are not encouraged in Chinese society. The Communist government, which since 1949 has actively promoted TCM as a cost-effective, efficient system of health care, has de-emphasized and suppressed much of its psychological and spiritual aspects. The government, focused on its ideological position of materialism, does not appear to value the psychological or spiritual. Consequently, in China, TCM is taught without emphasis on the complete integration of the spiritual and psychological elements that were basic and essential to the teachings of the ancients. However, given China's move towards globalization and a more democratic environment, and with the emigration of Chinese medicine doctors, I believe there will be renewed interest in TCM as it was taught centuries ago. I hope this renaissance will do justice to the original conception of Chinese medicine as a system of truly holistic scope.

For this reason, there is a general cultural reluctance in China to discuss emotional problems with a stranger, even with one's own doctor. A problem must not become an object of public shame, says one Chinese proverb. And as a busy surgeon in China, I had no time to discuss anything other than what was required to diagnose and treat my patients' physical problems, even if they had been willing to talk about their emotions.

During the first two years of my practice in Canada, women in particular talked to me about their depression and low self-esteem. Frequently, their "emotional" sickness was more debilitating than many of their physical symptoms, which puzzled me. I remember being struck by the words my patients used to describe how they felt: "depressed" and "tired" were overwhelmingly prevalent. I had no personal connection to these terms. In China, the word "depression" was not even in my vocabulary, and even though I worked long hours at the hospital, I don't remember using the word "tired" to describe how I was feeling. I was especially taken aback when I asked a little boy of six how he was. He told me he was tired. When I was his age, tiredness as a way of being was not part of my consciousness. Activity, fun and discovery filled my world.

I wondered if the strikingly similar emotional problems that patients presented were coincidences, or were part of a larger pattern. I was deeply concerned about how best to work with patients who presented emotional sickness. I consulted my peers and talked about returning to China for more training. I felt I needed greater knowledge to treat these patients, although several colleagues discouraged me from returning to China for further education. They felt that my medical background was solid, but that I lacked an understanding of the Western psyche and the accompanying psychological issues.

I decided to read more about Western psychology and to undergo psychotherapy myself. If I could understand how a psychotherapist worked with me, I would be in a better position to work with my patients.

Psychotherapy was a very different experience for me since, as a doctor, I had always been the listener. It provided me with

the first opportunity I'd had to really look at myself and understand the role that my unconscious played in my life. I discovered that much of my suffering was rooted in the events of my
childhood, when the expectations of my parents and culture had
weighed me down, and I struggled to be loved and accepted.

Therapy helped me to understand the pain that lies at the
heart of human suffering. The problems that we experience
are manifestations, to different degrees, of the deep fear, sadness, anger, worry, terror or obsession that lie within all of us.
As I recognized the causes of my own suffering, I also developed compassion for my patients' suffering. Though their
problems were different from mine, we shared in the pain of
our humanity.

My new perspective has had an enormous impact on my
own relationships. This is best illustrated by an experience I
had with a friend in China. Hua was becoming quite overweight, and my friends were worried about her. One of them
admonished her, in the direct, practical way Chinese friends
deal with each other, "Stop eating so much, don't be such a
pig. I love you and am worried about you." Hua replied, "OK,
I hear you, I'll stop eating." Though we were concerned about
the health of our overweight friend, we did not understand
the psychological and emotional causes of eating disorders.

When I returned to China not long after I began therapy,
my friends got together again, and we could see that Hua had
not lost weight. The others started ordering her to stop eating,
but this time I interrupted. "Don't yell at her," I said. "I think I
have a better understanding of why she's overweight." My
friends teased me, "Xiaolan's a fortune teller!" Later, when I
was alone with Hua, I asked her whether she was experiencing

marital problems. She told me that following the Cultural Revolution her husband had become a very successful businessman. Consequently, he spent little time at home, and their sex life was virtually nonexistent. She felt he no longer loved her. Because they were considered a perfect couple, Hua didn't feel comfortable talking about her feelings with anyone. She cried as she told me that she was starving for attention and affection. We discussed her deep feelings of rejection and how this might be contributing to her overeating. Perhaps she felt the need to create a reason—her unattractiveness—as a means to justify her husband's lack of tenderness and caring. Or maybe she was using the fat to create a physical wall to protect her from emotional pain.

Our experience together this time was very different from our last encounter five years earlier. Then, I would have joined my friends in trying to convince Hua to lose weight. Having learned about the importance of dealing with emotions, rather than somatizing them, I was able to see my friend differently, and talk to her about her loneliness and suffering. Learning about emotional health has also greatly enriched my practice. Although I've always known about the relationship between emotions and disease, it was from an objective point of view. With my own awakening to the interrelatedness of the emotional, spiritual and physical, the integration of the body, mind, emotions and spirit are even more integral to my practice. I hope this book will help you to rediscover aspects of yourselves that you can integrate into a healthier lifestyle.

NEITHER EXTERIOR NOR INTERIOR CAUSES OF DISHARMONY

The Neither Exterior nor Interior Causes of disharmony include diet, physical exertion and sexual activity.

DIET

An unbalanced diet can be the origin of disease, since it can promote patterns of disharmony in the body, and possibly disease. In TCM it is not so much a lack of nutrients that will disturb the body's balance as it is the types of foods that we consume too much or too little of. For example, too much salt can cause an imbalance in the Kidneys, leading to high blood pressure, water retention and headaches. Too many sweets may cause Dampness in the Spleen, leading to poor digestion, irregular bowel movements and edema.

Food can also be used as medicine in TCM—in fact there is an imperceptible line between the two. Shen Nung, who is regarded as the father of Chinese medicine, is responsible for the first Chinese herbal material medica, *Shen Nung Ben Cao*. More than 5,400 years ago, he classified herbs into three categories. Two of these categories comprise "medicinal herbs," integral in balancing the functioning of the Organ systems. The third category comprises "food herbs," which are part of our daily diet and consumed for strength, disease prevention and support.

Medicinal Herbs

Herbal medicine is an integral aspect of TCM and includes a wide range of plant extracts, as well as animal and mineral products, all sourced from the natural world. The therapeutic effectiveness of Chinese herbs is energetic as well as biochemical. Put another way, an herb is used that will energetically resonate with a specific Organ identified for treatment and biochemically affect it. This action will generate the smooth movement of Qi within that Organ system and thereby influence the other Organs as well.

Generally, TCM practitioners combine herbs to produce remedies that are specifically designed for a patient's unique constitution, emotional and physical health, and environment. This approach is in contrast to the Western medical model that prescribes a similar drug for a common condition based on research that demonstrates a relative degree of effectiveness of the medication on a select number of patients. In TCM, there could be fifty patients, each exhibiting the same conditions, but with very different underlying imbalances and constitutions. In this case, the doctor would prescribe fifty different herbal combinations, rather than one drug.

There are also, however, patent medicines in TCM, which are packaged herbal pills based on classical formulations. In China, manufacturers who meet rigid standards established by the government are allowed to produce these formulas. The disadvantage of packaged pills is that they are not specifically adjusted to address the particular needs of individual imbalance. The primary advantage of them is their low cost and ease of use, since preparing herbal remedies takes time and drinking them may be unpleasant due to their unfamiliar and peculiar taste. Moreover, patent pills are a convenient way to access the therapeutic power of herbs.

Food Herbs

The *Nei Jing* states, "If no food is eaten for half a day, Qi is weakened; if no food is eaten for a whole day, Qi is depleted." The food we ingest is of the utmost importance in supporting Qi and staying healthy. Dietary practices have been the basis for maintaining health and countering disease in the daily lives of Chinese people for more than 5,000 years. In general, we should eat moderate amounts of food, at regular times, according to our own hunger or thirst. But foods also have supportive characteristics that can promote or counteract patterns of disharmony.

One of the classifications of food is by flavour. As we learned in Chapter One, each food has a specific flavour that resonates with a particular Organ (see page 26). This is referred to as its "affinity," and allows the food's natural properties to act as healing agents for a particular Organ system. For example, sour foods, like vinegar and citrus fruits, are associated with the Liver; salty foods, such as celery and seaweed, with the Kidneys; bitter foods, like dark green leafy vegetables and bitter melon, with the Heart; sweet foods, such as yam and tuna, with the Spleen; and pungent foods, such as tofu and garlic, with the Lungs. At my clinic, treatment almost always involves some sort of dietary recommendation. If a patient has a weak Liver, for example, I will recommend that she eat more sour foods, such as lemon.

As well as being classified by flavour, foods are categorized by temperature: Hot, Warm, Neutral, Cool or Cold. These classifications do not only refer to their thermal temperature, but also to their energetic qualities. So barley, lettuce, tomato and duck are cold or cool in nature, while pumpkin, ginger, onions and chicken are hot or warm. If we are healthy and strong, we are more able to tolerate Hot and Cold foods. But if we are ill or feeling weak, we are more suited to Warm and Cool foods, such as chicken soup or orange juice. If one of my patients has a high fever, I ask her not to eat Hot or spicy foods such as cloves and cayenne pepper, which would only aggravate her symptoms. However, if a patient is internally "Cold" (a constitutional consideration that can only be diagnosed by a TCM practitioner), I suggest she eat more spicy foods.

Another consideration in maintaining balance through diet is climate. Cool foods, such as raw fruits and vegetables, tofu and rice, can be eaten when the weather is hot to release Heat. Warm foods, like root vegetables, lamb, and butter and cream, are good to eat when it's cold.

I remember farmers in China naturally adjusting their diet according to the season and their level of activity. When I completed high school, it was the middle of the Cultural Revolution (1966–1976), which was launched by Mao Zedong to eradicate traditional Chinese culture, customs and thought and supplant them with Maoist values and beliefs. Since Mao distrusted intellectuals, cultural objects and books that were representative of this group were destroyed and schools were closed. The upper and middle classes were stripped of their possessions and sent to labour camps in the country to learn from the peasants. I was given the choice between working as a farm labourer or staying in the city to work in a manufacturing plant. I chose to go to the country to be with my friends. As one of more than a thousand labourers, I lived in a one-storey farmhouse that consisted of a large room with twelve beds. The beds were grouped in six sets of twos with a mosquito net separating the adjacent sleeping cots. We each had a side table and a basin. Our kitchen/dining area was located in another building and our water supply was the well outside. Washroom facilities consisted of a building with crudely constructed stalls, each with a door that left the lower legs and head and shoulders of the occupant visible from the outside. Slats of wood arranged on the ground left a rectangular space open to the dug-out earth below. Here, we squatted to relieve ourselves. In warm months, our shower facilities were where we stood beside the well; during the colder months, we sponge-bathed in our dormitory, warming up the well water on the stove in the kitchen.

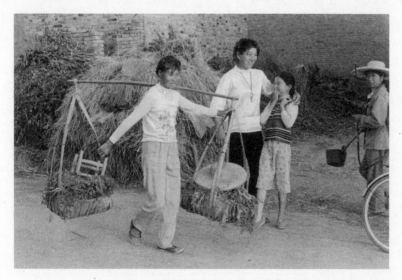

Harvest time on the re-education farm.

The farmers we worked for didn't usually consult doctors because of the distance to the city hospital and the cost of treatment. Instead they practised the self-care measures of Traditional Chinese Medicine. They adjusted their diets as they entered planting or harvesting times, eating more when they knew they needed the energy for the strenuous day of work ahead. Generally, during these periods, they would slaughter a pig and salt the pork to preserve the meat over the coming weeks. Then, during seasons when the crops required less tending, they reduced their food intake. They would have congee, or rice porridge, for breakfast with a few pickled vegetables, instead of a hearty meal of stir-fried rice, pork and eggs.

The time of year, the imbalances underlying our symptoms and our constitution are all contributing and interrelated factors in determining the appropriate therapeutic foods to eat. With this understanding of diet, we can include or exclude specific foods to prevent illness and maintain health. However, in determining the appropriate therapeutic foods for us, we need to be diagnosed by a TCM practitioner, who will make recommendations based on how our Organ systems are functioning. Transitioning from an unbalanced to a balanced diet must be gradual. Chinese medicine does not recommend a series of dietary practices that restrict what we can and cannot eat. It seeks to reestablish balance within the body, so that we can eat a variety of all foods in moderation, based on our own constitution, current health and climactic factors.

PHYSICAL EXERTION

Another cause of disease is fatigue, which can be the result of too much or too little physical exertion or work. Forceful and vigorous exercise, such as high-impact aerobics, commands the Qi and Blood to our muscles to sustain and support the activity, instead of fulfilling its role by circulating through the Organs of the body. Strenuous exercise continued over an extended period of time can exhaust Qi and Blood and lead to disharmony.

Though vigorous exercise may appear to alleviate symptoms arising from imbalances of Qi and Blood, it will not resolve them. The root causes of the problems must be addressed or we may come to rely on exercise for a sense of well-being, and this feeling of apparent good health will have detrimental effects. As well, strenuous exercise can injure or strain tendons, the tissue governed by the Liver.

At the same time, however, it is important to do a certain amount of physical exercise daily; otherwise, Qi and Blood become sluggish. If there is no physical exertion for an extended period, a Spleen Qi Deficiency will arise, resulting in cravings for sweets, weight gain, loose stools, excessive menstrual bleeding, muscle spasms and so on.

Time for sufficient rest, with care not to overwork or overtax the body physically, emotionally or mentally, is important for optimal health. The time spent for rest and for activity should reflect a balance that is neither too sedentary nor too demanding and draining, respectively. The primary way we get rest is through sleep. Since it is recommended that we spend up to one-third of our lives sleeping, it is important that we develop healthy sleep practices.

SEXUAL ACTIVITY

A lack of sexual activity can lead to disharmony in women. Orgasms promote the smooth flow of Qi throughout the Organ systems (read more on this in Part Four, "Clouds and Rain"). However, frequent pregnancies over a short period of time will deplete a woman's essence and shorten her life.

SUMMARY

A preventative, holistic approach to health care lies at the heart of Chinese medicine. Ancient Chinese philosophers advocated a science and philosophy—the Tao—to become

TABLE 4: BASIC CONCEPTS OF THE TCM APPROACH TO HEALTH

HOLISTIC	• The cause of a disorder is not necessarily located in the region of the symptom. Therefore our physiological irregularities, psychological factors and general character are observed to identify a "pattern of disharmony," which presides over any inquiry into cause and effect.
PREVENTATIVE	• TCM diagnoses and treats Qi imbalances before they become physical. • To prevent conditions from arising, we are encouraged to adopt a lifestyle and activities that are supportive to good health. • It is more beneficial to remedy an underlying problem than to adopt preventative measures so as not to produce new complications. For example, taking aspirin to prevent a heart attack (myocardial infarction) may cause a new problem—gastritis.
NATURAL	• TCM uses the natural healing forces of our body to help eliminate illness. • Symptoms of disease are not considered problems that have to be invasively corrected through surgery or drugs, but are viewed as signs that there is an imbalance that must be rectified.
FOUNDATION OF TREATMENT	• TCM identifies and treats a root cause of disease rather than treats symptoms.
FLEXIBLE TREATMENT	• Because symptoms are not pathologized with a universal treatment protocol, an individual, integrated view of symptomology, diagnosis and prescribed treatment are maintained.

aware of Qi, to control its flow and to live in harmony with the vital energy that is present in the human body and in the universe. By advocating a state of Yin Yang balance within the self, applied to society and the universe, Chinese medical texts taught the way to achieve health and thereby prevent disease. Living according to the Tao allowed the ancient sages to live very long lives. Table 4 summarizes some foundational aspects of the TCM approach to health.

Part Two

HEAVENLY WATER

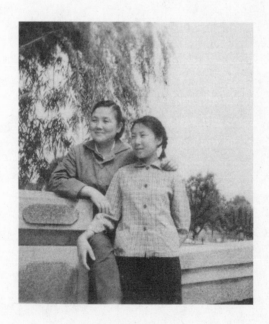

Me, age thirteen, with my mother

CHAPTER THREE

My Introduction to Heavenly Water

I first learned about the feminine cycle at the age of thirteen, in 1969, three years after the start of the Cultural Revolution. Though schools had been closed, China now entered a new phase, and young people were allowed to pursue an education. I had just started high school when my mother and father were finally allowed to leave the collective farm where they had been sent to work as labourers to atone for my father's position of authority as management at a television broadcasting station. My two older sisters and brother had also been away during this time as they, like all other former students, fulfilled their national duty to travel to Beijing to see Mao. As a result, I had lived basically on my own for two years, though I was often visited by family friends.

While it was a frightening and unsettling period in China, as children denounced their parents as traitors to Mao, and wives betrayed husbands, I have wonderful memories of spending time with my parents every day and sharing meals with them.

Food was scarce and rationed—we were each given monthly tickets for five ounces of meat and about twenty-five pounds of rice—but we were thrilled to be together.

I remember my mother gradually broaching the subject of puberty during this time. I knew something about it; I'd heard little bits of conversations at school about an "old friend" visiting and I'd read books that mentioned menstruation. These were not science texts, but novels. Though it had been forbidden to study books not written by Mao, I was an avid reader and had secretly read *Jane Eyre, War and Peace,* Charles Dickens's novels and many, many others, including banned Chinese classics. My friend and I hid them in our homes and brought them to each other, concealed under our clothes. One torrentially rainy day when my friend came to visit me, my mother answered the door and told him I was not home. When he turned to leave, she reached for his arm to bring him inside to dry off before venturing out again, and several books fell from under his coat. Mother was furious. She knew the Communists considered the possession of books—especially the classics—as grounds for incarceration. I was reprimanded severely.

The little I'd managed to find out about menstruation made me curious about it. I wondered how it would feel. My mother noticed me rubbing my breasts on occasion and asked if they felt itchy. She told me that I was growing up and developing breasts to feed a baby. She said that if my breasts felt a little itchy or painful, I should warm some vegetable oil on my fingertips and gently massage them.

My mother told me that soon I would be experiencing something "special" every month and that it was a sign I was maturing. With it would come new responsibilities. I had the sense that I was no longer supposed to be a naughty little girl, that I was to look after myself and be more considerate to others. My mother said that I would bleed from my vagina, and that it might be painful and I might feel nauseous, but not to worry; there were herbs that would help make my body strong and prevent any illness.

In preparation, she gave me a two-inch-high pile of sheets of coarse rice paper and a belt with a rectangular cloth strip that was connected to a string waistband. Attached to the cloth was a flap that looped over the string and fastened with a button. My mother showed me how to fold the sheets of paper into narrower strips and how to adjust the width for my comfort. When I wanted to change the paper pad, I would simply undo the button, remove the soiled paper and place clean sheets on the cloth. I felt a little embarrassed when my mother

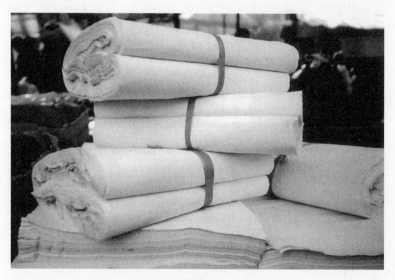

Rice sheets

explained all this to me. It brought into my consciousness the possibility of boyfriends, marriage and babies. Perhaps because I was a little slower in developing than my friends, I felt somewhat shy around this new phase of my life. But my mother told me it was all a natural part of growing into a woman.

The evolving feminine cycle was referred to in the *Huang Di Nei Jing* centuries before the birth of Christ and the Common Era. According to the *Nei Jing*, a woman's life comprises a series of seven-year cycles. At the age of seven years, a girl's Qi begins to thrive. By age fourteen, it should be strong and robust so that a girl can transform into a woman with the onset of menses. The body needs to be reassured that we are vital, that our Qi and Blood are at their fullest, before the start of an ongoing and regular loss of Blood.

Ancient practitioners called menstruation *Tian Gui*, or "Heavenly Water," because they believed that menstrual blood was different than the Blood that circulates through and nourishes our body. They knew that a man needed to ejaculate into the vagina for a woman to become pregnant, and that when she did conceive, menstruation would cease. Since they were not able to see the ovum with their eyes, they identified the reproductive Essence of the mother with menstrual Blood, equivalent to sperm in men. In his book on gynecology, *Fu Qing Zhu Nu Ke*, seventeenth-century Chinese gynecologist Fu Qing Zhu wrote, "Menstrual blood is not Blood but Heavenly Water, originating within the Kidneys . . . It is red like blood, but it is not blood. That is why it is called Heavenly Water." The *Nei Jing* states: "'Heavenly' indicates the descending of the True Qi of Heaven; 'Gui' indicates Water like heavenly clouds generating water." The Kidneys are where we store our Qi and our Jing (see page 28), or Essence, and are therefore responsible for our growth and development. Menstrual blood is not just a monthly discharge of discarded material from the Uterus. It is Essence, the vital energy that is needed to live.

The major component of menstruation is Blood. As taught by the ancient practitioners, menstrual Blood first begins to flow when a number of factors come together at the age of fourteen. Our Kidney energy must be strong and we have accumulated enough Blood to spill out from the Uterus. In addition, Qi and Blood are balanced and moving smoothly through the Zang-Fu Organs. And, the two Channels responsible for governing our seven-year feminine cycle must be properly functioning. The Conception Vessel (Ren Mai—the "Sea of all Yin") must be flowing strongly and the Penetrating Vessel (Chong Mai—the "Sea of Blood") must be abundantly supplied with Blood. When these variables come together, we begin to menstruate.

The start of Heavenly Water is a milestone in the feminine cycle. It is the beginning of the reproductive phase of our lives and marks a turning point in terms of our health. Because the onset of menstruation is a radical transition, it is a time of heightened vulnerability and must be supported with special attention and care.

With the start of my first period, I was able to eat special foods that I had watched my mother eat. For the five or so days when I was menstruating, my mother made a soup with eggs, raw cane sugar and homemade rice wine. The egg dish helps to increase circulation, nourish the body and keep it warm, thus aiding the smooth and free movement of Blood and Qi, and on the harmonious workings of our Zang-Fu Organs. Even my father knows how to make egg soup, and when he was aware that I was menstruating, he prepared the dish for me. It is common for Chinese men to have a good understanding of the foods that offer therapeutic value for women's health, and health in general, since prevention and treatment have been incorporated into, and are inseparable from, Chinese families' daily lives.

Egg Soup
Makes 1 serving

1 cup	water
1 tablespoon	raw cane sugar
2	eggs
3 tablespoons	rice wine

1. In medium saucepan, add 1 cup water and raw cane sugar. Bring to boil over medium-high heat.
2. Crack 2 eggs into boiling water, and bring to boil. Add rice wine and turn off heat. Serve hot.

My mother also cooked a sweet rice congee, a thin porridge with dried longan fruit, peanuts and red Chinese dates. The sweet rice helps the energy of the Liver to flow, the longan fruit activates the flow of Qi and increases Blood, the dates nourish Blood and invigorate the Spleen and peanuts also benefit the Spleen.

Sweet Rice Congee
Makes 4 servings

6 cups	water
1 cup	black sweet rice
1/2 cup	dried longan fruit*
10	dates
2 tablespoons	raw cane sugar
1/2-inch piece	fresh ginger, peeled and thinly sliced

1. In a large, heavy saucepan, add 6 cups water, black sweet rice, longan fruit, dates and raw cane sugar. Bring to boil over medium-high heat. Reduce heat and simmer for 2 hours, stirring occasionally. The finished congee will have the consistency of soup. Ladle it into a bowl and sprinkle with ginger slices.

At the onset of menses, periods do not occur on a regular basis, so my mother introduced me to *Wu Ji Bai Feng Wan,* or Black Chicken White Phoenix pills, to regulate my cycle. This patent remedy has been specially formulated to address general conditions related to Heavenly Water. My mother also suggested I rest, not lift heavy items or engage in strenuous exercise, and advised me not to drink cold water or eat cold foods, or to go swimming while I was menstruating. Because

---

* Dried longan fruit is available in Chinese grocery stores.

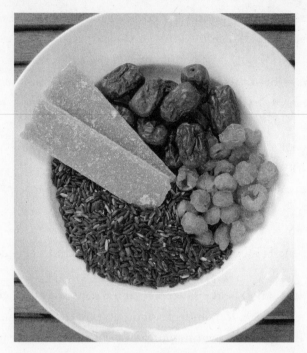

From the top clockwise, red Chinese dates, dried longan fruit,
black sweet rice and raw cane sugar

Blood flows outward from the Uterus during Heavenly Water, the body is in a state of Qi and Blood Deficiency—as Blood is lost, so is Qi. In this condition, we are more vulnerable to invasion by Exterior factors, like Cold. Ingesting cold foods or fluids during your period can obstruct Qi and suppress vital functions. Standing on a cold floor without shoes and socks when menstruating is another way for Cold to invade the body.

My patients often ask me what cold foods or drinks have to do with menstruation. I explain that the ingestion of cold or raw foods can tax and devitalize the Spleen. It is unable to fulfill its role to contain Blood within the vessel walls. When an imbalance occurs in our Spleen Organ system, we may

experience excessive bleeding, nausea, muscle spasms or cravings for sweets.

My mother was passing on to me what my grandmother
had taught her, what had been taught by the women through
the countless generations of my family. She was empowering
me to take care of myself through preventative measures in an
effort to optimize and safeguard my health. There is an intimate relationship between these dietary and lifestyle practices
and our menstrual health. Indeed, by following these recommendations, none of the females in my family experienced
any degree of menstrual irregularities.

CHAPTER FOUR

Harmonizing Heavenly Water

Our Heavenly Water depends upon the proper and balanced functioning of our Zang-Fu Organ systems and a smooth movement of Qi and Blood. Any disturbance—for example, tenderness in the breasts, headaches, irritability—during the time of Heavenly Water is cause for concern. These symptoms indicate there are imbalances in the body that, left unchecked, may progress to cysts, lumps, possibly tumours, and problems during conception, pregnancy, childbirth and menopause.

In the West, the collection of symptoms identified with the onset of Heavenly Water, such as bloating, cramps, tearfulness and so on, is referred to as premenstrual syndrome (PMS). I had never heard of PMS until I came to Canada. I was surprised to learn that in the West, the physical and emotional manifestations of imbalances in the body had been labelled a syndrome and were negatively associated with Heavenly Water. By giving these expressions of disharmony a name, our discomfort, pain and psychological suffering could be neatly dealt with—almost disregarded—by attributing our symptoms to PMS. It was clear that this significant time in our feminine cycle was considered a nuisance and a source of much distress.

Rather than grouping symptoms into a syndrome, Chinese medicine identifies patterns of imbalances within the Zang-Fu Organ systems. The syndrome known as PMS in the West is most often a pattern involving Stagnation of Liver Qi. The vital energy flow through the Liver Organ system has become stuck and cannot circulate properly. This is significant as the Liver is responsible for the balanced and smooth movement of Qi throughout the body. Since our emotions are manifestations of Qi, the Liver also regulates our emotions. And because the Liver regulates the flow of Blood, and Qi moves through the Liver network before it reaches the Uterus, the Liver also governs the menstrual cycle. Consequently, any emotional disturbances, such as irritability or feeling depressed around the time of our Heavenly Water, can be a sign that Liver Qi is blocked. When Liver Qi Stagnates, emotions get congested and there is an attempt to unblock the Stagnation through outbursts of anger or crying jags (tears are considered the fluid of the Liver). Since anger, resentment, annoyance and frustration are the emotions that are associated with the Liver, if it is out of balance, the possibility increases for us to feel these particular emotions more intensely and more frequently.

Because Blood is the vehicle for Qi, if there is a blockage in Qi, over time, Blood may also Stagnate, giving rise not only to emotional symptoms, but to physical ones as well. This has additional impact around the time of Heavenly Water, as the Liver stores the Blood that feeds the Uterus. Stagnant Liver Qi can manifest on a physical level as backache, tender breasts, headaches, feeling bloated, constipation, irregular periods, depression, breast masses and painful periods (dysmenorrhea). The Meridian through which Liver Qi moves starts at the inside of the big toes, ascends up the feet and the inner side of the legs. It goes to the pelvic region, where it encircles the Uterus, runs up the abdomen, then moves into the Liver and Gallbladder. It then travels up the front of the body, into the breasts, moving internally upwards to the throat and eyes (see Figure 5). That is why a Liver Qi imbalance can affect the lower abdominal areas, such as the ovaries, Uterus, fallopian tubes, Large Intestine, as well as the Spleen and Stomach Channels. The smooth movement of Qi through all these Organ networks is hampered, contributing to conditions such as breast lumps, emotional instability, abdominal distension, thyroid disorders, vocal dysfunction and heart problems.

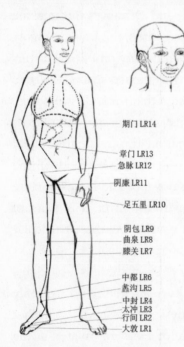

期门 LR14

章门 LR13
急脉 LR12

阴廉 LR11

足五里 LR10

阴包 LR9
曲泉 LR8
膝关 LR7

中都 LR6
蠡沟 LR5
中封 LR4
太冲 LR3
行间 LR2
大敦 LR1

Figure 5: The Liver Meridian

The accumulation of Blood Stasis in the pelvic area restricts the flow of Blood to the ovaries and Uterus. This can result in blood clots, cramps, fibroids in the Uterus, infertility, pain during intercourse and cessation of the flow of Heavenly Water (amenorrhea).

Stagnating Liver Qi and Blood are generally a result of suppressed, unexpressed or excessive emotions. Since the Liver is the Organ system that maintains an intimate relationship with the emotions, it is the most prone to problems of constraint, congestion and Stagnation. In my clinic, I see women weekly who have lost their Heavenly Water due to unexpressed emotions that they are unaware of or unable to give voice to. The emotion may be guilt, which was what Jane experienced after the death of her mother. Jane was thirty-eight years old when she came to see me. As I worked with her, Jane told me how her single mother had come to adopt her. Her mother was one of her best friends, and Jane was immensely grateful for her love, acceptance and help. The two of them decided to go on a trip together and started making plans. Unfortunately, Jane was forced to cancel due to work commitments. Her mother decided to go on without her, and while she was away, was killed in a car accident. Jane plunged into despair, where she moved between grief and guilt. She couldn't forgive herself for not accompanying her mother on the trip, and her regrets weighed heavily on her. Eventually, Jane lost her period and her hair began to fall out. It was at this point that she came to see me.

Knowing that her feelings of loss and guilt were blocking her Qi, I talked with Jane, allowing her to express her deepest feelings. She told me about her childhood and how her mother took care of her, and made her feel wanted and special. I encouraged Jane to write about her feelings in a journal, to document the time she shared with her mother. Integral to her treatment was the release of the feelings that were gripping and constraining her Liver Qi and Blood, stopping the flow of her Heavenly Water. Jane expressed her profound sadness and guilt in her journal and gradually came to terms with her feelings. Her period returned and her hair stopped falling out.

One of the times in my life when my emotional health had a dramatic impact on my Heavenly Water was in 1988, after my immigration to Canada. I had left China to pursue a post-graduate degree in pharmacology at Queen's University in Kingston, Ontario. My knowledge of the English language was very limited and I arrived in this small Canadian city knowing no one. I found a room in a house close to the university, which I shared with another student and my landlord. I didn't cook or eat meals at the house because I didn't have cooking equipment or dishes. I was also seldom home because I left by seven-thirty in the morning and returned home around ten at night. I spent each day attending classes and studying English in the library, where I would listen to my lecture tapes over and over again. I ended up eating convenience foods like peanut butter and cookies; they were perfect for sneaking into the library. My landlord also taught me to make sandwiches, so my diet consisted primarily of simple foods like these, and not complete, balanced meals.

Nearly every night I cried as I missed my family and friends and China. I was really feeling the difficult position that I had placed myself in. I would fall asleep listening to my English tapes; in fact, I was plugged into my cassette player for so long that the inner part of my ears became sore and chafed from the earphones being pressed against them.

Christmas of that year will always remain an unpleasant memory for me. The university had opened one section of the library for students like myself who had no place to go for the holiday. When the library closed at six o'clock, it was already dark and very cold. I walked the few blocks to my rooming house. When I arrived, the front door was locked, and I realized I had left my key in my room. All the shops and restaurants in the city were closed and it was too cold to sit down, so I decided to walk around the block. I walked once, twice, three times and kept walking, counting my steps and listening to my tapes. I wanted to cry but was afraid that my tears would freeze on my face. Fortunately, I was dressed very warmly and did not feel cold as long as I was moving. I felt as if I was in a dream and that this wasn't really happening to me. One hour after another passed, until close to midnight my landlord arrived home and opened the door. I fell into bed and for a short while my body shook with sobs. But I was so exhausted, I quickly dropped into a deep sleep.

My Heavenly Water flowed the first month I was in Kingston, but after that it stopped. I was shocked because my cycle had always been so regular, a constant in my life. I went to buy Black Chicken White Phoenix pills, but unfortunately, they were not available in Kingston. I asked my parents to send them from China. In the meantime, I massaged the area below my navel to encourage the Blood to flow. I finally received the pills from my parents, but the impact of the depression and stress on my Liver Organ system stopped the movement of my Heavenly Water for eight months.

Women in the West sometimes find it hard to believe that their relationship with their emotions, particularly anger, resentment, frustration and irritation, could have such a direct impact on their menstrual health, but emotional and mental problems are powerful origins of imbalances in the body. If the mind is not at rest, Qi becomes overactive, and if there is constant irritation, Qi can get obstructed and stuck. Understanding how we can work with the emotional, physical and mental aspects of ourselves and bring them into balance has far-reaching influences on our menstrual health and overall well-being. Because of the mutual dependence of all the Organs, the anger that hurts the Liver, or the fear that injures the Kidneys, or too much joy that distresses the Heart, or the anxiety that harms the Spleen, or the grief that damages the Lungs, will each produce an imbalance in the other Organs over time. The emotions are expressions of energy, so their smooth and regular movement ensures good health.

If we are having problems with our Heavenly Water, the first step is to take stock of how we are feeling, get in touch with the emotional stresses and worries that block us, and then work to free ourselves from them.

SHARON

Sharon had never experienced any problems around the time of her Heavenly Water. However, when she began to realize that the child she had hoped for was not going to be conceived with her husband, she began to suffer from cramps, bloating, tender breasts and other symptoms associated with PMS. Her husband was not interested in having children and wanted to return to university to pursue yet another degree. Sharon had been the breadwinner for most of their married life. Though she loved her husband, she felt it was unfair that the child she longed for was not going to become a reality. She was angry but didn't express this to him. "I was scared to rock the boat,"

Sharon told me. "I didn't know how to confront him . . . I had no model for working through this. I came from a traditional family and did what I thought I was supposed to—stay with him through thick and thin."

Sharon's anger turned inward and she became depressed. Her feelings were intense, but she didn't know how to express them. She had some understanding of her problems but didn't know how to deal with them. Sharon started to see a counsellor, began sitting with a meditation group and threw herself into her work. Over the next seven or so years, her menstrual health declined. Her periods started earlier and earlier, her cramping was more severe, her breasts were sore more often, her bloating continued. She said, "I didn't do anything about it because I thought everyone had this. I thought it was normal."

Sharon's life with her husband narrowed so dramatically that they only went out with each other. He had to be the centre of attention and would often undermine her. She continued to suppress her feelings, and her self-esteem eroded. "I never did anything in public or with our families that would contradict him or could be taken as a criticism," she said. "I didn't do anything that would cause him to lose face or embarrass him. Basically I kept my mouth shut."

Sharon began experiencing periods that were extremely heavy, alternating with trickling flows. Her cycles became irregular, beginning eight days after the end of her last period. Her breasts were sore in the middle of her cycle and the cramping was very painful. Sharon's abdominal bloating was so severe that someone asked her if she was pregnant. Her doctor told her that she had two cluster fibroids in her uterus that, combined, were the size of a sixteen-week-old fetus. Fortunately, they were benign. The doctor said that the fibroids were a result of high levels of estrogen, that her body wasn't producing sufficient progesterone.

Sharon began using a natural progesterone cream. She also began an aggressive self-care program. She read up on supplements and eliminated red meat, processed food and dairy products from her diet. An exercise regime Sharon adopted included yoga, low-impact aerobics and muscle conditioning. She also began to see a deep-trance channeller. He encouraged her to look at herself physically, emotionally and spiritually, and helped her to get in touch with her anger. She began to understand how terrified she was to face her marriage, but she bravely resolved to seek counselling with her husband.

Less than a year later, Sharon decided to leave her marriage. She said that until that time, "I was taking care of him. Now I can remember who I am." Once her husband had moved out of the house, Sharon began to clear out all traces of him. For the first time in almost two decades she felt joyous when she awoke. She said, "I had given my power away and I was taking it back."

Within one month of her separation, Sharon's doctor gave her the happy news that her fibroids had shrunk by half. For Sharon there is no doubt about the powerful causal relationship between her suppressed anger, her irregular periods and the development of her fibroids.

Sharon had a lot of support and continues to work with someone who helps her connect with what she wants and believes in. He was instrumental in helping her recognize what she was afraid to see and then to handle what arose. Social or professional support plays an important role in helping alleviate emotional stress. Sometimes the reasons for our stress are not apparent to us, and talking to someone can help us become aware of the reasons. Often we can better deal with upsetting emotions and traumatic life circumstances by talking with professionals or confiding in trusted family members or friends who can help us resolve our problems. Many of us try to deal with our disturbing emotions on our own, but will be pleasantly surprised at the relief and well-being we feel when we share our feelings, thoughts and experiences with others. By doing so, we come to identify what exactly distresses us, become aware of the intensity of our reactions and understand what meaning we give to them. We may come to see how this hinders us in generally moving forward in many aspects of our lives and health.

If you are not inclined to share your feelings with others, then the use of diaries, or journaling, is a therapeutic way to express yourself. Writing a journal is for your own health, so record your innermost feelings and deepest thoughts. By documenting our feelings, we become less identified with them. Journaling creates space so that we can separate ourselves from our negative feelings. Consequently, we give ourselves the opportunity to see ourselves with fresh eyes and make different healthy choices. Moreover, writing about our feelings allows us to transform them and move towards better feminine health. If you feel too busy or stressed to write, it's probably time to pull out your journal, sit down and put pen to paper—or fingers to the keyboard. Journaling, however, should never become another onerous task. Rather, it should help reduce your emotional burden.

CATHERINE

Often it is a long and painful process to uncover the root cause of our symptoms around Heavenly Water. For Catherine, it was a journey that crossed the Atlantic Ocean several times and brought her excruciating pain almost two weeks out of every month for over two decades.

At the age of fourteen, Catherine experienced such intense pain in her abdomen that she was hospitalized. The severe pain was her introduction to Heavenly Water, although she wasn't told this at the time. She had no understanding of menstruation, as her mother and two older sisters had not told her what would happen to her during her cycle. Catherine had no idea that this racking pain would reoccur regularly. The following month Catherine experienced pain so great for the seven to ten days prior to her period and for three days at the beginning of her flow that she was taking painkillers and drinking brandy to bring some relief. Her mother told her she had "the curse." In rural England where Catherine lived at the time, this was a term often used to describe menses. Catherine's mother also suffered from menstrual pain, but since Catherine was not aware of "menstruation," she had no idea that she and her mother shared this experience.

Two months after her first period, Catherine and her family moved from England to Toronto. For Catherine, this was an incredibly difficult transition. In moving from a village of approximately two hundred to Toronto, a city of about two million at that time, Catherine experienced a great feeling of displacement and loss. Even though she spoke English, her accent was so different that to others it sounded like another language. And she lost the countryside and hills, where she often sought solace from the village and her family.

Catherine's pain spread from her abdomen throughout her body, and now extended four to five days into her period. After a year and a half of living in Canada, she was diagnosed with rheumatoid arthritis in her left arm. When Catherine was sixteen, a doctor offered her a suggestion to alleviate her pain—he recommended she have a baby! Two years later, Catherine was prescribed oral contraceptives to ease her pain. After three years, she developed severe headaches. When she asked her doctor if it was safe to take painkillers and the birth control pill, the medical practitioner expressed surprise that the oral contraceptive had not brought relief of Catherine's menstrual symptoms. She was made to feel that her pain "was the way it was" for women, and that it was her responsibility to accept the situation.

Catherine graduated from university and began working in the publishing industry. She continued her regimen of painkillers to feel "comfortably numb" while her pain progressively intensified. She was passed over for promotions at work because of her frequent absences. Catherine was feeling increasingly isolated in her pain. After working in Canada for a year and a half, she decided to move back to England, where she felt more at home.

Two years after returning to Britain, Catherine realized that the distension that often accompanied her pain was not limited to the time prior to and during her flow. It was now occurring every weekend! She was checked for endometriosis (a disease where the tissue called endometrium, which lines the uterus, grows in areas other than the uterus), fibroids, polyps and cysts. She underwent a laparoscopy, a surgical procedure that uses an instrument similar to a miniature telescope to bring light into the abdominal area for direct examination. As Catherine awoke, she was shocked to see blood coming out of her navel. The doctor told her, "There is absolutely nothing wrong with you." She suggested that Catherine have her digestive system checked out.

Ten days after the laparoscopy, Catherine still wasn't able to go to work. When she returned, there were rumours that she had taken the time off to have an abortion. Catherine was given increased responsibilities at her job along with a commensurate title change, but she did not receive the raise she had been promised, and the announcement of her new role was never circulated within the company. It was at this point that she decided to quit her job. She found a part-time position, a short walk from her home. For four months, Catherine's routine was to work in the morning and sleep from one in the afternoon until six, rise for something to eat, and go back to sleep until the next morning. During this period, Catherine decided to return to Canada. It was also during this time that she decided to see a homeopath recommended to her by a friend who worked in a health food store. She had had the name for about six months but was reluctant to call; she had been conditioned to believe that homeopathy was "wacko and a form of quackery."

On her first visit, the homeopath took her history and asked Catherine what she wanted. She replied that she wanted to be well before she returned to Canada, and was prepared to do whatever was needed. After giving her some homeopathic pills that brought Catherine to laughter and then tears within minutes, the homeopath asked her if she could see the pattern of loss in her life. The homeopath's words resonated deeply.

This powerful experience started Catherine's three-month radical homeopathic treatment. She worked with the homeopath and had many, many dreams and nightmares, cried what seemed like endless tears, not always knowing what her sadness was about, and slept. Slowly her life was unravelling. She began to realize that others had denied what she was feeling. And the more her reality, her feeling world, was squashed and ignored, the greater her pain.

Catherine's return to Canada was the start of an intense spiritual journey. She attended a workshop in guided meditation, and while others felt as though they were floating in the clouds, she felt like she was drowning. She then went on a spiritual retreat during which she experienced a psychic unwinding—she could feel the healing energy opening in her hands. Her old paradigms around mind, body and emotions were shattering and she was embarking on a path to become more conscious of ways to understand her pain and her life. Catherine met people who helped her become conscious of past life traumas she'd experienced, and who showed her ways to deal with them. Her memories centred on children, mothering and motherhood, torture, rape and dishonour. These experiences were poking holes in her reality. She felt as if all her coping mechanisms were disintegrating.

A couple of years after her return to Canada, Catherine's pain was still excruciating, but had shortened to one to two days prior to her period. Also, the area of pain had shrunk, and as she brought more memories to the surface, pain related to that memory decreased, then disappeared. Catherine was discovering that when she was able to embrace a memory, she experienced less pain. Now that she had a new understanding of the relationship between her mind and body and emotions, she made an agreement with her body: if it provided her with one piece of information, she would take medication to alleviate the pain.

After three years of consciously abiding by this agreement, she had a momentous breakthrough: she was able to remember being raped at the tender age of three years old! This was an extremely significant element of her healing. Pieces of her life started to fit together. She remembered making a conscious decision, at age eleven, that she wanted nothing to do with being a woman. Growing up in rural England, she saw women being dishonoured and violated. At this young age, she rejected the denigration of the perceived feminine. In doing this, she was denying her sense of womanhood. With the memories that surfaced, Catherine now had a more profound understanding of what lay at the root of her desire to separate from being a woman. She began to see how denial was robbing her of her feelings; the more she denied her emotions, the greater her pain.

As she became more in touch with her feelings, her rheumatoid arthritis disappeared. Today Catherine no longer takes pain medication. Giving time and space to connect with her feelings has reduced her pain to an area around her right ovary. As Catherine remembers who she is, her pain lessens more and more.

Catherine's journey to the root of her menstrual pain is one that has involved a great deal of courage and commitment. As she said, "I followed my inner knowing." When we can do this, we can trust in our process of emotional and spiritual unwinding, and find the source of our physical pain. Sometimes, the origins of our symptoms reside external to our inner worlds, in places we could never consciously imagine.

Women who experience significant pain during the time of Heavenly Water are often prescribed oral contraceptives. Birth control pills are also prescribed to regulate menstrual periods for those women with excessive bleeding (menorrhagia) or for those whose Heavenly Water has stopped flowing (amenorrhea). In TCM, birth control pills are said to cause Liver Qi Stagnation. The conditions and symptoms that arise may manifest while you are on the pill, and even later on in life.

SANDRA

Sandra was a twenty-eight-year-old woman who was referred to my clinic by a doctor of Western medicine. At age thirteen, she experienced excruciating cramps during the time of her Heavenly Water. Her doctor prescribed birth control pills to alleviate her menstrual pain. Now, fifteen years later, she visited her general practitioner because of the discomfort and pain she experienced during intercourse. Her doctor examined her, then tested her hormone levels. The horrifying results were returned: Sandra was experiencing the onset of menopause! After discussing her options with her doctor, Sandra decided against hormone replacement therapy (HRT). She was concerned that by taking HRT as a means of dealing with early menopause, she was opening the door to myriad unknown complications, such as the possibility of ovarian or breast cancer. When Sandra came to my clinic, she was unsure of what approach to take. She was also concerned about her fertility. After treating Sandra with acupuncture, Tui Na and herbs for approximately six months, the pain she experienced during intercourse started to subside, and her Heavenly Water began to flow again.

When Liver Qi cannot flow freely, Blood cannot move to the Uterus and over time may Stagnate. Blood Stasis can give rise to infertility. In China, women typically do not take oral contraceptives until after the birth of their only child (a one-child policy was established in China in 1979 to restrict population growth). They are concerned that artificially increasing hormone levels may affect their capacity to conceive by creating a condition of Liver Qi and Blood Stagnation. In Sandra's case, the Western medicine treatment of her symptom with birth control pills gave rise to more complicated and serious problems: early onset menopause, possible difficulties in conception and severe pain during sexual intercourse.

The severe menstrual cramping that Catherine and Sandra experienced represents one of the many symptoms, in addition to those classified as PMS, that can manifest at the time of Heavenly Water. The major underlying root of these irregularities can be traced to the Causes of Disharmony (see pages 30 to 45). Specifically, these include emotional strain, but also exposure to Exterior pathogenic factors that invade the body, irregular diet, overwork and excessive physical and mental exertion. Due to the intimate relationship between the Organ systems, each of these factors also plays a crucial role in the weakening of Kidney Qi.

The Kidneys are the other Organ system that, when out of balance, is a major cause of symptoms related to PMS. Kidney Essence, in originating Heavenly Water, plays a major role in reproduction, growth and development, as well as pregnancy and childbirth. Deficient Kidney Qi will manifest as long-standing fearfulness that results in premenstrual water retention, lower abdominal distension, back pain, reduced libido and urinary tract infections, connected with the time of Heavenly Water.

CHAPTER FIVE

Our Relationship with Ourselves

One of the worst famines in history took place in China, from 1959 to 1960. I vividly remember my grandmother's legs swelling to double their size, as her protein intake dramatically decreased. The protein deficiency caused Kidney system complications that affected her water balance, causing extreme fluid retention in her legs.

In my clinic in Canada, I spoke with a woman whose swollen legs looked remarkably and frighteningly like my grandmother's. Moreover, she had lost her Heavenly Water. I discovered that because she was afraid of gaining weight, she was restricting her diet to a minimal amount of brown rice and water each day. This highly educated, professional woman exhibited the same symptoms as my malnourished grandmother, but for very different reasons.

Prior to my coming to Canada, the concept of skinny as beautiful and desirable was foreign to me. In the West, many women try to develop what the media tells them are perfect bodies. In China, I was taught that a woman's beauty is reflected in her intellect and heart, and the way she takes care of herself. Healthy, bright, good-hearted women were the ones considered beautiful. Perhaps because when I was living in China, Chinese people were generally not overweight, there was no connection between beauty and weight. Or perhaps the connection was negligible because of the absence of an aggressive and powerful advertising and marketing engine promoting the concept of the perfect woman.

In Canada, I've met many women who seek validation based on an idealized standard of beauty. I have heard them speak of feeling disempowered due to their physical attributes. I have witnessed their poor body image and low self-esteem affect the flow of their Heavenly Water. It is distressing to see women of normal weight and shape struggling to adhere to yet another extreme diet, or exercising maniacally to lose weight. I tell them, "You look beautiful," but they aren't able to hear my words, and if they do, they don't believe them. I have seen ten-year-old girls struggling to lose weight and am profoundly concerned at the impact of this activity on their fragile psyches, and the repercussions of severe dieting and strenuous exercise on their growth and menstrual cycle. Their eating habits have become distorted, as they opt for fast-food binges or an extreme reduction in their overall intake of food. Eating disorders among today's female adolescents and young women are epidemic. Though they are intelligent and seemingly successful in many facets of their lives, they have an extremely unhealthy relationship with food and their bodies.

Our relationship with our bodies deepens during the time of Heavenly Water as we experience radical changes. How we relate to our physical form has a profound effect on how we value ourselves. I remember my mother telling me when I was a young girl that it was normal for a woman to have a tummy bulge, that this was beautiful. Soft round curves were a natural part of the female body, she said. Neither my family, friends nor the society I grew up in placed emphasis on my physical appearance. Instead, the focus was on how I conducted myself, what I was like as a person, how I interacted with others. When a Chinese man of my generation or older sees a woman considered beautiful by Western standards, he sees an idealized view of beauty that he "can look at but not eat." He separates a woman he would like to marry from an ideal that is fun to behold. In his view, a physically beautiful woman does not make the best marriage partner. Instead, he considers the qualities of loyalty, trust and commitment priorities in selecting a mate. (This, of course, may be changing as China becomes more exposed to Western culture.)

When I came to Canada in 1988, I wasn't concerned with my physical appearance in the same way as Western women are. I did not feel any connection between my self-worth and the way I looked. Rather, I based my self-worth on my academic achievements, my ability to succeed at whatever I undertook, my health and my physical strength and endurance. But after living some years in Toronto, I started saying I was full even though I wasn't. At the time, I didn't think much about my motivation. Then a close friend asked me why I was eating so little, and as we talked I realized that I wanted to lose weight! I had been absorbing the rampant media messages about the relationship between thinness and beauty. I was taken aback that I, who was so aware of the dangers of listening to these messages, had ended up unconciously getting caught up in them. This experience made me appreciate the tremendous pressures that both women and men experience as they are continually bombarded with unattainable standards of beauty and norms of acceptability. I now have a greater understanding of the insidious, subliminal nature of media images. It is so easy to incorporate standards of beauty into our psyches without being aware we're doing it. But we're affected emotionally by our feelings of acceptance or rejection, and we're affected physically when we try to alter our bodies to fit unhealthy ideals.

CHAPTER SIX

Self-Care During Heavenly Water

Since disturbances in Heavenly Water are principally rooted in the Liver and Kidney Organ systems, we should undertake self-care treatments that support these networks. In general, we can best tend to our Heavenly Water by working with our emotions, making dietary changes, moderating our physical activity and making other lifestyle changes. Keep in mind that because being relaxed is very important to the smooth movement of Qi and Blood, any self-care regimen we undertake should be with gentleness and not approached aggressively.

DIET

In general, and especially during the time of Heavenly Water, excessive amounts of cold foods and fluids, and raw foods, should not be ingested since they can hamper the transformation process of food into Essence—Jing—one of the Three Treasures. Cold foods can slow down the work of the Spleen, and lead to Spleen Qi Deficiency, which hinders the flow of

Qi in the body and, if prolonged, can create accumulations of Cold and Dampness. This deficiency will produce pain, perhaps in the joints, which is a frequent problem for us during the time of Heavenly Water, and may increase bloating, cramping and discomfort. In addition, the Spleen ensures that Blood stays within the vessels and does not seep into the tissues, so the Spleen's proper functioning is important during menstruation. A Spleen Qi Deficiency can manifest as heavy menstrual flow, cramps with cold hands and feet, diarrhea and digestive problems. When a Spleen Qi Deficiency results in a Blood Deficiency, we may have problems falling asleep or miss a menstrual period.

What should we eat to prevent Qi deficiencies? Foods, even slightly cooked, are more easily digested, with nutrients more readily absorbed. Hot drinks and soups help to alleviate painful periods. On the other hand, coffee, alcohol, hot and spicy foods, along with large amounts of red meat, should be avoided during Heavenly Water, as they Stagnate the free movement of Liver Qi. Since the Liver Meridian courses through the Uterus, a blockage here will affect the smooth movement of Qi and Blood, and create uncomfortable symptoms. Generally, stimulants magnify disharmonies of Excess and increase the severity of symptoms.

Rich, fatty foods affect the free movement of both Liver Qi and Spleen Qi. Typically, oily foods that are fried or greasy, and sweets, can produce Spleen Qi Deficiency, and so should be avoided. A high-fat diet increases Qi Stagnation and Dampness, which is related to depression and loss of energy. Additionally, not eating an excessive amount of dairy products and raw foods will reduce Dampness and not tax the Spleen.

During the time of Heavenly Water, women frequently experience a craving for sweet foods. One theory suggests this is a sign of a Spleen Deficiency. Another theory relates it to the Liver Organ system. As the Liver becomes full, it exerts its inherent assertive quality, while the Spleen, fatigued from transforming and transporting digestibles, is weakened in its ability to fend off aggressive advancement by the Liver. Generally, it is thought that the Spleen is weak and needs support, thus explaining food cravings as a Spleen Deficiency. However, the cause may be an aggressive Liver that, susceptible to excessive Qi, tends to become full prior to the start of menses due to stress and emotional disturbances. A Liver with excessive Qi will result in the weakening of the Spleen and cause increased desire for sweet foods. Some women crave chocolate and coffee. The caffeine temporarily moves stagnant Qi but does not address the root problem and ultimately has a rebound effect, causing a deeper level of Stagnation and Spleen Defiency.

Salt intake should also be reduced to ease its effect on the Kidney Organ system. Salt, in excess, can create a Kidney Qi Deficiency that may result in water retention, lower-back pain or urinary tract infections.

To replenish Blood that is lost during Heavenly Water, we should eat foods that are rich in Blood-enhancing properties such as dark green, leafy vegetables like spinach, kale and dandelion leaves, and red meat, liver, poultry, sweet rice, fish, eggs and raisins. It is also beneficial to eat the egg soup and sweet rice congee (see pages 56 and 57) that my mother taught me to make. Whenever one of my staff experiences some menstrual discomfort, I encourage her to stop working and prepare the egg soup.

PHYSICAL EXERCISE

Mary was an athletic thirty-two-year-old woman who had gone through some milestones in her life. She had recently married and also graduated from law school. Now, she and her husband wanted to have a baby, but they were concerned because Mary's periods came so sporadically, perhaps four times a year. She was extremely thin, with a very straight silhouette. I remember saying to her, "I'm not sure where a baby can grow, you'll first need to put on some weight."

When I prescribed herbs for Mary to take, she expressed concern that they would make her gain weight. Mary's preoccupation with her weight was driving the quality of her health and possibly her ability to conceive. She was exercising strenuously daily to remain thin and fit. But the profuse perspiration that accompanies vigorous aerobic exercise results in a loss of fluid that can drain Qi and cause a Blood Deficiency, which in turn has a negative effect on the flow of our Heavenly Water. This is the reason that many female athletes experience menstrual irregularities or lose their periods (amenorrhea). Another symptom that Blood is not flowing properly is hair growth in atypical locations, since hair is connected to Blood. Mary, for example, had abnormal hair growth on her chin. After treating her with herbs, acupuncture and Tui Na, Mary's periods became regular.

Qi and Blood must be relaxed in order to fill the Uterus, then overflow as Heavenly Water. Hence, strenuous physical exercise is not recommended during menstruation. At the onset of menses, excessive exercise can have a negative impact on the menstrual health of pubescent girls. Since the body-mind is undergoing radical changes at this time, activities that nurture balance are needed. Balanced activities will also help girls develop a more positive body image and enhanced self-esteem.

When I worked on the farm in China, I was always given a three-day leave when my Heavenly Water started to flow. It was standard practice for all the young women workers to be relieved of heavy physical work during menstruation. The Chinese perspective on the significance of the time of Heavenly Water is evident in a 1997 survey of Chinese labour law, published in the *Asia Women Workers Newsletter*. It states that women who are menstruating cannot be assigned "work at high altitudes, low temperatures, or in cold water, etc." In addition, a large number of companies in China have internal policies that grant a two-day leave to a woman during menstruation.

QI GONG AND TAI CHI

A very effective way to support Qi is to practise the ancient Chinese art of Qi Gong or Tai Chi, both of which are orchestrated dances of breathing and movement, combined with meditation, that restore the flow of Qi and Blood along the Meridians and reestablish harmony in the Organ systems and the body as a whole. In practising these ancient arts, we become aware of Qi and learn how to regulate its flow. The exercises engage the body in movement (Yang) and allow for quiescence of mind (Yin), leading to a state of enhanced physical health and mental relaxation. In this way, Qi Gong and Tai Chi attune our Three Treasures: Jing, Qi and Shen. They nurture our vital life-force energies to prevent disease and promote health, long life, physical strength and spiritual growth. They can also help in the treatment of many conditions and diseases by stimulating the natural healing capacity of the body.

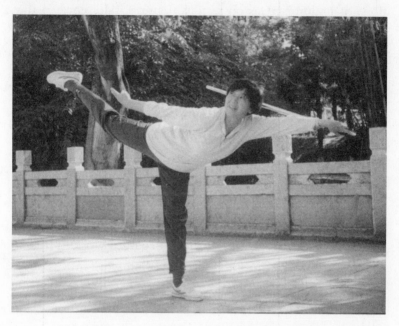

My sister Xiaoping practising Tai Chi in Kunming

A doctor of Western medicine introduced Lisa to Qi Gong. He suggested she might be interested in this practice as a means to work with her stage-four endometriosis. "I had this disease for ten years," Lisa said, "although I couldn't get clinically diagnosed until I had surgery. A decade ago, I had what's called a chocolate cyst, discovered by ultrasound. It is an accumulation of old blood that is typical of endometriosis. Gradually my periods got worse, the cramps intensified . . ."

Laparoscopic surgery is the only definitive means for Western medicine to diagnose endometriosis. Around the time Lisa was scheduled to have the procedure, she met her husband and moved to the United States. She cancelled her surgery. At this point she had no understanding of the implications of endometriosis on fertility. Later, Lisa discovered that many infertile women may be afflicted with endometriosis.

Lisa returned to Canada and once again booked surgery. However, fortunately for her, within one month of deciding to try to have a baby, she conceived. Two and a half years ago she gave birth to a son. "I had no idea," she said, "of how lucky I was to get pregnant with endometriosis. And then after the birth of my son, I wasn't sure what to expect. Often, endometriosis can subside after childbirth." Lisa's endometriosis didn't go into remission, but she had several months without any pain. At first her life was wonderful—it felt complete.

A few years ago, Lisa's husband began to work in Russia. He would spend a month in Canada, then work in Russia for a month. Lisa was alone about 60 per cent of the time. They tried to find a location that would reduce his commute and allow them to spend more time together as a family. She knew they needed to make a decision but found it difficult to do so. Lisa's stress increased. As her stress escalated, so did her pain. She described it " . . . like labour. It felt like contractions. The pain was no easier to deal with. I was incapacitated, I couldn't function." She had cramping some months, and a period that was irregular. At this point, Lisa began to take painkillers.

Over an eighteen-month period, Lisa's pain increased so that she was suffering for more than half the month. Her pain was reeling out of control, and her medication was no longer adequate to manage it. Even though she didn't want surgery she visited her surgeon. "What do you do for yourself?" he asked her. Lisa replied, "Acupuncture, massage, yoga." He said, "These mostly involve other people helping you. What do you do yourself?" It was at this point that he mentioned Qi Gong. She was familiar with the martial arts, and Tai Chi, and didn't think this form of exercise was for her.

On a return visit, Lisa was told that she had a 4 $1/2$-centimetre cyst on her left ovary. Within a matter of weeks, it grew to 6 $1/2$ centimetres. She and her doctor decided to go ahead with the laparoscopy. The cyst was growing at a rate that was extremely dangerous; there was a high risk that it would rupture. Lisa wanted to conceive again, so was focused on preserving her fertility.

In an effort to support her body before surgery, Lisa began an intensive treatment of acupuncture three times a week with me. She also began meditating and doing guided visualizations. She had a live-in housekeeper to help her with the domestic tasks, and she devoted her time to what she most wanted to do—be with her son. Her mother came to stay with her when her husband was away, and Lisa also found a babysitter to help her look after her son. She did her best to continue a normal life. "Lying back and experiencing my pain," she said, "was worse than going about my life." Lisa continued to focus on reducing her stress and pressure. She said, "I know now that when I was under stress it affected my cyst."

At one of Lisa's preoperative appointments, she mentioned to her surgeon that she was seeing me, a TCM practitioner. He pulled out an application for a workshop being offered by a Qi Gong master the week after her surgery. At the last minute, Lisa decided to attend, but there was no space available.

Lisa's cyst did not rupture and she was positively diagnosed with endometriosis. When she awoke from surgery, her doctor said, "OK, we found a spot for you in the workshop." As the anaesthetic was wearing off, Lisa had been babbling about Qi Gong. Having heard this, her surgeon made some calls and arranged for her to attend. "[Going to the workshop] was a life-changing experience," she said. "The clouds lifted over me. Literally, from the first exercise, my body was moving without instructions. It was doing what it wanted to do. We were told to 'smile from our hearts.' When someone asked how they were supposed to do this, the master replied, 'Don't think about how to do it, just do it.' Everyone was encouraged to let go, let whatever needed to be released, be released."

I asked Lisa how she would describe Qi. She said, "Qi is the energy in every cell. Everything is made from energy. Think of Qi as the energy that makes the world go round. It makes blood move through the body, it makes the trees grow, it brings gravity to earth." Lisa continued to practise Qi Gong. "I learned three exercises that I repeat for about 15 minutes a day. Since I took the workshop I have experienced an over-whelming sense of joy and less abdominal pain. I'm not doing Qi Gong to cure my endometriosis. It clears my mind, and some days are better than others. Qi Gong makes me feel good and I see it as a way to become a better person."

Qi Gong and Tai Chi cultivate our bodies through physi-cal movement and develop in us acute mental awareness. We can also engage in regular meditation to nurture our insight. With a consistent meditation practice that can be as simple as breathing exercises, we can cultivate the mindfulness and clar-ity to deal with our emotions in a healthy way. Through meditation we develop the equanimity to accept the unsatisfactory circumstances of our lives with compassion and loving kindness.

Thich Nhat Hanh, a Vietnamese Buddhist monk, learned to transform his anger at the injustices he'd witnessed in his country during the Vietnam War through a practice of mindful breathing and walking. Mindfulness is an intensified awareness of what we are experiencing and what is happening around us in the present moment, without censorship or criticism. When we are able to be in the here and now, we are less attached to our agendas and can more readily flow with what is brought into our lives. When we breathe in, we know that we are breathing in, and when we breathe out, we know that we are breathing out. When we lift our foot to take a step, we are aware that we are lifting our foot. When we are angry, we are aware that we are angry. This objective noticing allows us to obtain a new perspective on our anger. Mindfulness allows a "witness" to develop that enhances our attention and the meaning of our experience. By making anger the focus of our attention, witnessing removes the "charge" of the anger, and all the habitual (conscious as well as unconscious) responses that typically accompany it.

Considering that one interpretation of Qi is "breath," a practice focused on the breath can also help to sustain and stimulate Qi. Breathing exercises are not so much about doing something as about becoming aware of the breath and allowing it to occur naturally. The following is a breathing exercise that can be done sitting, standing or lying down:

Take a deep, slow inbreath, expanding your belly. Exhale deeply, contracting your belly. Now watch your breath: Is it fast or slow, shallow or deep? Are you holding your breath? Are you fully exhaling? Can you feel the breath on your nostrils? Is it more apparent on the inhalation or the exhalation? Is your abdomen rising and falling, is your chest rising and falling? Do certain people cause you to hold your breath? Is there a difference in your breathing when you are walking, sitting, standing or lying? Allow your breath its own rhythm. As you pay attention, you may notice the qualities of your breathing change—just follow it and notice what is happening. This exercise helps us to become aware of our breath, our Qi, and also naturally helps reduce tension and stress that can obstruct the smooth movement of Qi.

HERBS

When I worked on the farm, all the girls with whom I shared a dormitory knew which herbs to take to support us during the time of Heavenly Water, and we had the opportunity to pick them fresh in the country. I remember going for walks after dinner with my workmates, strolling along the edge of the dusty road. We'd often go out, not necessarily for exercise, but to alleviate the feelings of missing our family and friends and the fear that this kind of life was all that the future held for us. As we walked, we would see *Yimu Cao*, an herb that is part of the grass family, growing in the ditches. This herb is well-known for its ability to help tone the Uterus, which is a muscle as well as an Organ, and so requires toning. During the time of Heavenly Water, if the Uterus is not strengthened, there is an increased possibility of menstrual irregularities, such as excessive bleeding, scanty flow or cramping.

On our walks, we'd pick *Yimu Cao* for each other and take it back to the kitchen to make a tea with it, by boiling the grass in water. Often, we'd gather more than we needed and would dry it by hanging it upside down for the times when we were too busy for a walk or when it was not the season to harvest it.

The use of herbal remedies was so incorporated into our daily lives that each of us knew the herbs that would support us during the time of Heavenly Water. We did not need our mothers to remind or cajole us to take herbal remedies that would prevent menstrual problems and promote health. This self-awareness was part of our upbringing as Chinese women.

There are two patent herbal remedies that can be found in Chinese herbal shops in the West that are very effective for regulating Heavenly Water. One is the remedy my mother introduced me to: *Wu Ji Bai Feng Wan*, or Black Chicken White Phoenix pills. They offer a broad range of safe applications. By enriching Blood and strengthening Qi, this medicine treats abdominal pain, vaginal discharge and sore breasts. The pills can be taken three days prior to the start of a menstrual period to three days after the flow of Heavenly Water stops. The dosage and frequency varies according to the manufacturer.*

The other herbal formula, called *Xiao Yao Wan* (pronounced "shao yao wan"), is effective in smoothing the flow of Liver Qi and nourishing Blood and Spleen Qi. The pills will relieve pain from menstrual cramps and ease emotional

---

* Check with your doctor before beginning use of herbal medicines if you have allergies, drug sensitivities or any serious illness like heart disease, high blood pressure, diabetes, epilepsy or glaucoma; or if you are taking any prescription medications. Stop taking the herb and call your doctor if you experience any of the following symptoms within two hours of taking it: nausea, diarrhea, headache or vomiting.

distress, irritability and mood swings. This remedy can be taken daily, according to the manufacturer's directions for up to six months, with great benefit.

SELF-CARE TREATMENTS

There are a number of other measures we can take to care for ourselves during the time of Heavenly Water. First, use sanitary pads rather than tampons. Blood and Qi move downwards and out when we are menstruating, and tampons block this natural flow. Also, if we experience heavy bleeding, the Blood can move backwards, resulting in Blood Stasis, or old Stagnant Blood not being eliminated. If Blood becomes obstructed in tissues, it can produce lumps and masses such as ovarian cysts and uterine fibroids or, in some cases, endometriosis.

It is important to maintain balance between work and rest. Engaging in an extended period of work, whether it is physically putting in long hours of work or mentally working overtime, will deplete Kidney Qi. Moreover, the accompanying physical strain that arises from sitting or standing too long can weaken the body's vital energy. If we sit at a computer for an extended length of time, the strain on our eyes will also affect Liver Qi, since the eyes are the sense Organ associated with the Liver. When we maintain a body posture over a prolonged period or work at an intense pace, we don't have time to replenish ourselves, and end up consuming our Essence, the precious overall energy that we received from our parents. The depletion of Essence will result in a Kidney Qi Deficiency that will hinder the Kidneys from performing their responsibilities in reproduction, development and growth. Having too many demands placed on us also increases our stress and affects the flow of our Liver Qi.

To reduce the prevalent Western disorder of sleep deprivation and the accompanying emotional stress, maintain a regular sleep schedule. Also, try not to eat before you go to bed, and abstain from stimulants such as coffee, alcohol and cigarettes that can affect your sleep. Additionally, the *Nei Jing* states that we should change the time of rising and retiring according to the season. In the summer, we should get up early and go to bed late, while in the winter, we should get up late and go to bed early. In doing this, we will resonate with the Yang energy of summer and the Yin energy of winter.

If you have painful periods, massage the lower abdominal area with warm castor oil. If applying heat relieves the cramping, you can also mix together 30 grams each of ground cloves, cinnamon, ginger and *ai ye* (dried mugwort) and put the mixture in a small cotton pillow, roughly seven by seven inches. Warm the pillow in a microwave or in a cast-iron frying pan over low heat until it is warm to the touch. Do not allow it to get so hot that it burns your skin. Place the pillow on your abdominal area. This remedy can also be used for back pain. A heating pad might also help ease the discomfort.

Treating and managing pain is an important step in self-care. From a Chinese medicine perspective, pain is the red flag that warns us of Stagnant Qi or Blood. It can generally be dealt with by getting in touch with our feelings, or by expressing our emotions, or by finding our voice to be heard, or on a more physical level, through topical preparations, diet, exercise and rest.

ACUPRESSURE

Acupressure can also be very helpful in supporting the Kidney Organ system. Apply firm pressure in a downward motion with the thumb or knuckles to the following acupressure points:

YONG QUAN

On the sole of each foot, between the second and third toes, approximately one third of the distance between the base of the second toe and the heel, there is a depression below the ball of the foot. This depression is the acupressure point Yong Quan, and is sometimes referred to as "Bubbling Spring." Massage this point with strong pressure directed inwards and towards the big toe. Slight discomfort or mild pain when you do this indicates a blockage. Apply pressure for one minute. (See illustration below.)

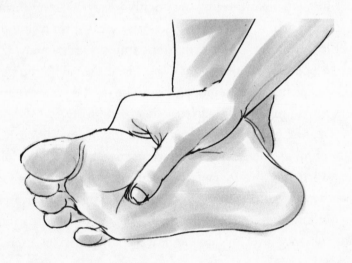

SAN YIN JIAO

This point benefits the flow of Spleen, Liver and Kidney Qi, and is located on the inside of the lower leg, approximately three finger widths above the ankle. Apply pressure to this point by moving your fingers or knuckles in a kneading motion twenty times. This is one of the most important acupuncture points to benefit Heavenly Water. It is the juncture point of the Spleen, Liver and Kidney Channels. It can balance the Spleen; promote the Spleen's function of transportation of water to drain Dampness; sedate the Liver so it will disperse Liver Qi; and support the Kidneys. Massaging this point can help relieve feelings of irritability, engender calmness and alleviate pain in the abdominal area. (See illustration below.)

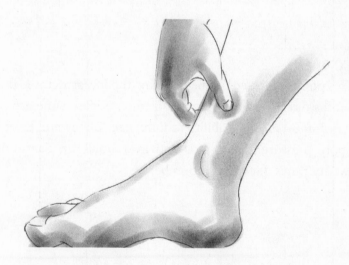

ZU SAN LI

On the outside of the leg, approximately four finger widths below the bone that protrudes just below the knee, is a point that can be massaged to balance Spleen Qi and nourish Blood. Knead it twenty times. (See illustration below.)

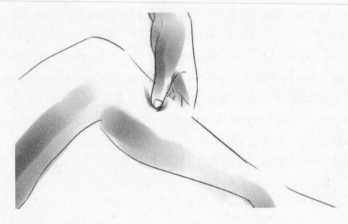

NEI GUAN

This point is located on the inside of the forearm, three finger widths directly above the wrist in the middle of the arm. It's very important in its ability to influence Kidney and Liver Qi. Apply pressure downwards and in a small circular motion twenty times. (See illustration below.)

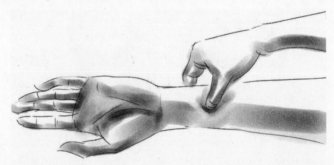

SUMMARY

In terms of Heavenly Water, it is primarily our relationship with our emotions that is most critical to health. In Chinese medicine, emotions are a manifestation of Qi, our vital life force. When the movement of Qi is impaired, illness or disease can occur. Blood and Qi are also intimately interrelated, and so imbalance in one often results in dysfunction in the other.

This notion of relationship and interconnectedness resonates throughout Chinese medicine. The TCM practitioner takes all aspects of our being—physical, emotional and spiritual—into consideration when making a TCM diagnosis. Conditions are not treated; rather, therapeutic remedies are recommended based on a holistic view of the person. Moreover, the treatments themselves are holistic and customized to the patient. The treatment of premenstrual abdominal distension, for example, would include suggestions for dealing with anger and frustration, as well as recommendations for diet, lifestyle, exercise, rest and work. Balance is sought in all aspects of life.

Although gynecological disorders can be traced to any Organ because of the interrelationship of the Organ systems, it is primarily the Liver and Kidney Organ networks that are responsible. The Liver stores the Blood that is forwarded to the Uterus for discharge, and the Kidneys provide the Essence that is required to supply the Uterus with Blood and Qi for the normal flow of Heavenly Water.

For women, the primary self-care treatment is to deal with emotional disturbances. Other recommendations include: dietary therapies, including herbs, regulating exercise regimens, Qi Gong and Tai Chi, meditation, self-massage and lifestyle considerations.

Looking after our feminine health requires that we maintain a close relationship with our natural physiology. We must be aware of the subtle and not so subtle shifts that occur, which may be the precursors of disease. In addition, if we can see how our health depends on the activities we engage in daily, the emotions we express, the attitudes we maintain and the food we ingest at every meal, we may become more closely connected with the functioning of our bodies and feel empowered in moving ourselves towards health. Chinese medicine gives us hope that we ourselves can prevent illness and facilitate health.

SELF-CARE RECOMMENDATIONS
- Stay in touch with your emotions, and find ways to constructively express them.
- Maintain internal harmony and peace.
- Eat foods and herbs that support the body and prevent illness.
- Work towards a balance between work and rest, physical and sedentary activity.
- Use self-massage to stimulate the flow of Qi.
- Dress according to the weather.

EMOTIONAL HEALTH
- Talk to someone about your feelings (a friend, family member or TCM practitioner).
- Develop awareness of when you are denying your emotions.

- Learn your stress/emotional triggers.
- Keep a journal.

DIET

- Avoid eating excessive amounts of coffee, alcohol, red meat, hot and spicy foods.
- Avoid excessive consumption of dairy products.
- Avoid eating excessive amounts of greasy, fried and sweet foods.
- Do not consume large quantities of salt.

During the flow of Heavenly Water

- Do not eat cold foods or drinks, or raw and frozen foods.
- Eat dark, green leafy vegetables, such as spinach and kale, and sweet rice, fish, eggs, raisins, liver and poultry.

RESTORATIVE PRACTICES–SPIRITUAL

- Qi Gong
- Tai Chi
- Meditation

LIFESTYLE

- Avoid excessive work.
- Maintain a regular and balanced schedule for eating, sleeping, working, exercising and resting.
- Dress appropriately for the weather.

During the flow of Heavenly Water

- Avoid swimming.
- Do not lift heavy items.
- Do not engage in strenuous physical activity.

- Avoid the use of tampons.
- Do not walk around in bare feet on cold floors.
- Do not engage in sexual intercourse.

Part Three

LOTUS BLOSSOMS

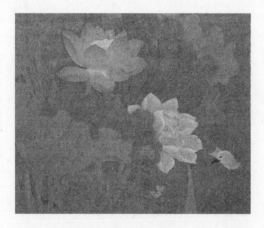

Lotus and Ducks, late thirteenth-century Chinese
painting on silk (detail)

CHAPTER SEVEN

Caring for Our Breasts

Our breast health, like our Heavenly Water, depends on the smooth flow of Qi and Blood through our Zang-Fu Organ systems. Within the breasts, a number of Meridians pass through: the Liver Meridian, the Kidney Meridian, the Stomach Meridian and the *Chong Mai,* or Penetrating Vessel, which originates in the Uterus and branches out in tiny vessels throughout the breasts. A blockage in the flow of Qi and Blood within any of these Meridians can therefore cause

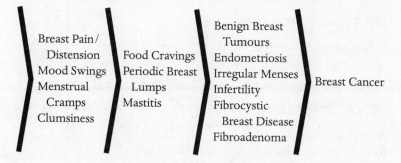

Breast Pain/
Distension
Mood Swings
Menstrual
Cramps
Clumsiness

Food Cravings
Periodic Breast
Lumps
Mastitis

Benign Breast
Tumours
Endometriosis
Irregular Menses
Infertility
Fibrocystic
Breast Disease
Fibroadenoma

Breast Cancer

Figure 6: Continuum of Breast Disorders

Stagnation in the breasts and lead to a continuum of progressive breast disorders that may begin with premenstrual breast distension and over time evolve into more serious diseases, including breast cancer. Figure 6 shows the steps along the succession of breast conditions that can arise from progressive Stagnating Qi and Blood.

Breast tenderness or lumps will not inevitably lead to breast cancer, nor will the order of symptoms occur exactly as indicated in Figure 6. The reasons that one woman's symptoms will manifest as breast pain and another's as breast cancer are attributed to the severity, complexity and the duration of the imbalance. Having a history of benign breast lumps, however, is considered a significant risk factor for breast cancer, since the root cause of both conditions is the same. Stagnant Liver Qi is the primary cause of most breast problems, and premenstrual breast distension and benign breast lumps may be part of the evolution of a Liver Qi Stagnation that may progress to a carcinoma. Therefore, diagnosing and treating Liver Qi Stagnation is an effective way to prevent a more critical disease, and there is much we can do ourselves to support our breast health.

SELF-CARE MEASURES

While Liver Qi Stagnation is the leading cause of breast conditions, insufficient Kidney and Stomach Qi, and Stagnation in the Chong Mai, can also lead to imbalances in the chest area. Self-care measures, therefore, focus on smoothing, balancing and promoting the flow of Qi within all these Organ systems to help reduce the risk of breast disorders.

EMOTIONS

As discussed in Chapter Four, emotional distress is the biggest factor in hindering, taxing and impairing the flow of Liver Qi. Ancient practitioners wrote that the emotions are the most significant cause of breast disease. The seventeenth-century text *Fu Qing Zhu Nu Ke* states: "Depression injures the Liver, pensiveness affects the Spleen, accumulation develops in the Heart, the channel-Qi stagnates and generates nodules."

One of the very few women whom I knew in China who had breast cancer was a successful forty-five-year-old doctor who was married to a renowned physician. When I spoke with her, the overwhelming topic of discussion was her marriage. She told me of her husband's adultery and the emotional abuse he inflicted on her. She found her marital situation extremely depressing but felt trapped, since divorce was not an option she felt she could consider. Her Heavenly Water, she told me, had become abnormal in timing and flow a few years prior to her diagnosis, and she had experienced stabbing pain in her breasts. Her life force was not vital, it felt stagnant and, in fact, she said that dying would be a better alternative than continuing to deal with her life. She looked as if she was gradually being eroded by her husband's abuse.

Unresolved, chronic or excessive emotions can damage or impair the Liver Organ system. If the Liver cannot move Blood easily because of a blockage in the flow of Qi, Blood may become sluggish and Stagnate in the breasts, the area through which the energetic pathways of the Liver traverse. So our feelings of well-being play a profound role in the health of our breasts. We should not subdue or hold back our emotions, nor should we explosively express them without awareness and restraint. Critical to our health is how we validate, appropriately express and accept our feelings and emotions.

When I lived in China, the incidence of breast cancer was low, relative to what I subsequently witnessed in the West. Since the primary origin of breast disease is attributable to emotional stress, what is the difference between the West and the East in terms of emotional stress? Could the difference in breast cancer rates be a reflection of Chinese women's ability to resolve their emotions? Or is it because Western women experience different emotional stresses? In a typical Chinese medicine response, I don't believe there is any one explanation. I think a complex web of different factors are at play, such as the level of stress in Western society versus that in the East, how we are culturally conditioned to deal with emotions and, for lack of another term, our philosophical contexts.

It has become apparent to me as I have developed my clinical practice and made a life in Canada that stress is a pervasive aspect of Western culture. There are many variables, influences and decisions that I need to consider in living my life. Where will I live? Should I buy or rent? Where should I work? What is the best way to conduct my clinic for my patients' healing? How do I find good staff? What is it that I ultimately want to do to help the most patients? How might I accomplish this? What is the most effective way to resolve or deal with a volatile emotional situation? We have a lot of choice, which inevitably is accompanied by a lot of stress, as we are faced with myriad daily decisions. In fact, having so many choices is in effect similar to having no choice, since we often feel paralyzed, overwhelmed, not knowing how to make an appropriate decision.

Many women talk to me about their desire "to do" something with their lives, but are unclear as to what this might be. They consider the many options available to them, they weigh the pros and cons, and as they do so, other possibilities surface. This further compounds the initial choices and options they must deal with. Deliberation becomes the focus, and fear of missing out on a "better" alternative or making a "wrong" choice renders them helpless, making them feel disempowered to take action or make a commitment.

In China, my career was decided for me. My personal hopes, wishes and dreams were not taken into consideration. At the end of my time at the collective farm, we were told that a number of us would be allowed to pursue an education. I desperately wanted to study but was afraid to compete with my friends for the privilege. Nevertheless, I applied and was chosen. Growing up with a father who worked in broadcasting and a mother who expressed herself articulately through the written word, I was greatly interested in journalism as a profession. Writing allowed me to connect with people by capturing emotions and thoughts that they may have been unable to put to words. However, my dream was not to be realized. I was informed that I would be going to medical school. I would become a doctor. Upon completion of my studies, I was assigned employment at a hospital, and came to understand what was expected of me. Choices around my career were virtually nonexistent, but I was happy to have a career, and I feel very grateful that being a doctor has proved to be fulfilling and rewarding.

In China, where one lived was based on one's employer. Housing options were connected to the company or government department where one worked, as well as the level of position one held. Each company had apartments that were allocated as part of the terms of employment. In general, decisions pertaining to work and accommodation were not within the average person's sphere of influence. I'm not suggesting this was a good situation, but the emotional strain that accompanies increased personal choice is not present in Chinese society—at least not yet, to any significant degree. This, however, is bound to change as the economic and political situation in the country changes.

The way in which Chinese people express and deal with emotions is culturally determined. Confucianism, with its specific codes of conduct, still exerts a dominant influence on Chinese behaviour. Social harmony is considered of the utmost importance and is achieved through proper and understood roles and responsibilities towards family and others. Other contributors to harmony are the restraint of emotions, conformity, and compliance and subjugation to authority. Taoism echoes the Confucian ideals of emotional calm and conformity, along with an emphasis on the mystical elements of human nature. Other cultural determinants are an emphasis on "face." Losing "face" or dignity through "wrongdoing" brings tremendous shame to the individual and family involved. This is deeply ingrained in Chinese people and has the power to direct actions and words. As a result, Chinese people are restrained in expressing their emotions, concerned about the overall harmony within the group, and have a tendency to associate emotional difficulties with physiological imbalances. Perhaps for Chinese people, there is little sense of psychologically needing or having to work through feelings since these are considered manifestations of body disorders.

Additionally, there isn't a strong sense of emotionally striving for what they want or need, since first, personal choice is not an ingrained part of the culture, and second, individual needs are subordinate to the needs of the family or group, and society in general.

This cultural outlook affects the way Chinese people deal with their emotions and live their lives. Since emotional disturbances are the major source of breast disease, this cultural conditioning, combined with the comparatively lower degree of stress the Chinese experience due to their limited choices, may help to explain why Chinese women have the lowest rates of breast cancer in the world, while Western women have the highest. Having said this, however, external factors such as diet, lifestyle, environment and so on are also reasons why Chinese women are much less apt to develop breast cancer. Though these factors are not considered as significant as emotional health, they nonetheless can offer support in attaining health.

DIET

A diet that supports the free flow of Liver Qi is beneficial in preventing breast disease. Conversely, it is important to avoid or minimize dietary factors that hinder, tax or impair the flow of Liver Qi. If Liver Qi is sluggish, there is a tendency for it to slow down, become constrained and produce Heat, since Qi is inherently warm. There are specific foods such as hot, spicy, peppery or fatty foods, along with excessive amounts of red meat and alcohol, that contribute to the accumulation of Liver Heat. These foods, along with chocolate and caffeine, are also stimulating and Heat-producing, and should be eaten in moderation since they aggravate the Liver. Foods that overly excite Qi upset the balance between Qi and Blood by drawing Qi to the surface of the body. This creates problems for the Liver in ensuring the smooth flow of Qi and Blood throughout the system.

A healthy Spleen/Stomach Organ system can prevent the Liver from becoming blocked and imbalanced. If the Spleen is weakened, Liver Qi may Stagnate and be in Excess. Since cold, frozen and raw foods, greasy foods and dairy products can contribute to Spleen Qi Stagnation, we should not eat too much of them. These foods tend to lead to the formation of Dampness, or the accumulation of fluids. Dampness hinders the Spleen's ability to transform and transport fluids, and may result in the formation of Phlegm, one of the key contributors to the development of breast masses.

Generally, we should eat a well-balanced diet with adequate amounts of a variety of foods. It is important that we eat moderate amounts regularly, since over- or under-eating can either tax the Spleen in its ability to extract Food-Qi or result in the production of insufficient Food-Qi. The former scenario will lead to a weakened Spleen and the latter to Deficient Qi and Blood.

EXERCISE

We should all engage in moderate exercise. Practising Qi Gong or Tai Chi (see page 86) is an effective means of regulating and promoting the flow of Qi and Blood within the body. There are many different forms of Qi Gong and many, many different exercises. Qi Gong can also be combined with Tai Chi movements, meditation, relaxation and breathing exercises.

LIFESTYLE

It is important to prevent exhaustion before or during the flow of Heavenly Water. We should restrict physical as well as mental exertion, as excessive and prolonged fatigue can exhaust Qi and damage the Chong Mai. Sluggishness in the flow of Qi and Blood in the Chong Mai is a major factor in the development of breast masses.

RISK FACTORS

In addition to a history of breast conditions, several other risk factors increase the chances of developing breast disease. These include:

AGE

Because the Chong Mai originates in the Uterus and branches out in tiny vessels throughout the breasts, the cessation of our Heavenly Water, or menopause, may result in Stagnation of Qi and the formation of breast congestion, tenderness and masses.

Additionally, the Spleen's ability to transform digested food into Qi decreases with age, often resulting in Deficient Qi. With insufficient Qi to move Blood, Blood may Stagnate and eventually accumulate in specific areas such as the chest or lower abdomen. This may lead to Blood Stasis, one of the key factors in the development of breast lumps.

FAMILY HISTORY

A family history of breast disease may be closely linked to the similar lifestyle choices family members make. Certain learned dietary habits and responses to emotional disturbances can be factors in the development of breast disorders.

EARLY OR LATE MENARCHE

The start of the flow of Heavenly Water at too young or too old an age is considered a possible factor in the development of breast disease, since it may indicate excessive Liver Qi. The start of menarche is closely connected with the development of the breasts, and an excess in Qi may lead to premature budding of the breasts.

NOT GIVING BIRTH

During pregnancy and childbirth the Uterus houses the fetus and then discharges the baby. In so doing, it purges Stagnant Blood and Qi, fulfilling a deep, cleansing function. If we put off childbirth or do not give birth, then old Blood and Qi are more inclined to accumulate. Initially, this may lead to Stagnation in the Liver system in the lower region of the body, the pelvis, that may then also congeal in the breast area as the Stagnation progresses over time.

CHAPTER EIGHT

Possibilities at the Upper Branch of the Continuum

A tumour is not the root cause of breast disease but the "upper branch" of the illness. Because breast tenderness and a benign breast lump are both part of the evolution of breast disease that may progress into a carcinoma, the self-care measures given in Chapter Seven should be followed whether you have breast pain or you have been diagnosed with a malignant tumour. Of course, women who have breast cancer must also decide between various treatment options.

Ancient practitioners differentiated between the ability to treat malignant lumps, which they referred to as *Ru Yan*, or "breast stones," versus benign lumps, which they called *Ru Pi*, or "breast nodules." In the Yuan dynasty (AD 1281–1358), Dr. Zhu Dan Xi wrote: "Worry, anger and depression cause accumulation, Spleen-Qi is weakened, Liver-Qi free flow fails, there is a hidden nodule formed like an egg without pain or itching; after several years, it forms an ulcer and it is called *Ru Yan*." He acknowledged that breast stones were more difficult to treat than breast nodules. Because the stone is a hardened mass, it is more dense and generally takes longer to disperse than an imbalance that is not as solid.

Western medicine treats breast cancer through radiation, chemotherapy, hormonal (anti-estrogen) therapy and surgery, and breast cancer survival rates are higher than they've ever been. TCM treats breast cancer through herbs, acupuncture and Tui Na to balance Yin and Yang in the body, detoxify the Liver system and support Kidney energy. Though Western and TCM treatments are often successful, there is no treatment that is absolutely guaranteed to cure cancer.

Women who are diagnosed with breast cancer are generally fearful and uncertain about what course of treatment they should pursue. I have seen that the process in making the decision is a critical one. Understanding the pros and cons of their alternatives, and allowing whatever it is they need to feel empowered to make this decision, is crucial to a woman's healing. When I am asked to explore options with my patient, I will consider her age, her family history, her personal and dietary habits, how long she has been aware of the lump, the size of the lump, the location of the lump, whether or not there is discharge from the nipples and the colour of the discharge, the shape of the lump, whether the surface of the lump is smooth or irregular like a cauliflower, and the degree to which the lump is mobile. Then I will confirm my diagnosis with the results of a biopsy. There are so many variables at stake when making an informed decision, but one of the most important aspects of doing so is to feel confident in that decision and to be unequivocally supported in it by family, friends and medical practitioners. Making a decision about treatment with support and love allows a woman to be in an active relationship with her illness. This facilitates healing and allows a woman to live with her illness, thereby providing the material, mental and emotional basis for dealing with it.

Some women decide to pursue all treatment options available to them. They may have radiation and chemotherapy and also see a TCM practitioner to help them deal with the side effects of the treatment. Other women decide that certain treatments are not for them. I have some patients, for example, who decide not to have chemotherapy because of its possible side effects. These women sometimes come into censure from their families as a result, and this disapproval can make them feel hesitant or guilty, or cause them to regret their decision. These types of emotions can negatively impact the flow of Qi through the Liver Organ system—a system that is already taxed. Emotions have an enormous impact on a woman's ability to fight cancer. It is important to try to remain optimistic, to look on the bright side and to never give up.

The philosophical basis and roots of Chinese culture may provide a helpful way of understanding illness and dealing with its emotional aspects. Two fundamental philosophical perspectives in China are Yin and Yang, and Buddhism. In the concept of Yin and Yang, the universe is continually changing, moving and transforming. All phenomena and events are in a relationship, which involve opposing but complementary forces that are under the influence of universal energy. This means that everything has two sides, and a healthy state exists when the two forces are in relative balance. There can never be a state where there is only sadness or only happiness. They exist in relative balance or imbalance with each other, and each is necessary for the other to exist. Happiness is not necessarily a feeling that must exist exclusive of sadness. Happiness and sadness must coexist, since the roots of happiness may be found within sadness, and to be happy carries with it the seeds of sadness.

There is a Taoist parable that expresses the relative nature of opposites: One day a farmer was telling his neighbour about his horse that ran away. The neighbour sympathized with the farmer, saying, "That's too bad." The farmer replied, "You never know what is good or bad." The next morning the horse returned. But it was not alone. It brought with it many wild horses. The neighbour said to the farmer, "Congratulations, it's good that your horse has returned and brought many other horses." Again the farmer said, "You never know what is good or bad." The next morning the farmer's son went to mount one of the wild horses. The horse threw the young man, who fell off and broke his leg. Once again the neighbour sympathized with the farmer. For the third time, the farmer said, "You never know what is good or bad." The next day soldiers rode by. They were forcing young men to join the army. Because of his broken leg, the farmer's son was not conscripted.

Like the neighbour in the story, we have a tendency to want to make things absolute—good or bad. This desire for a fixed, infallible ideal is at odds with the Chinese concept of Yin and Yang, which is based on a relative ebb and flow rather than a fixed idea that is static. A shift from the latter perspective results in a very different way of interacting with the world and with life. It is often referred to as a "both and" perspective, rather than an "either or" view. What this means is that each of the events that happened in the parable are *both* good *and* bad.

This concept of Yin and Yang has far-reaching implications for how meaning is given to our emotions, as well as to illness. In the West, illness is viewed as the "enemy" to be conquered. There is an emphasis on biological "cure," in which health triumphs over disease. From the point of view of Yin and Yang, this notion of an exclusive state of health without disease is not possible, since well-being and illness coexist. Good health reflects a balance between the two states, while disease is a manifestation of disharmony in the flow of Qi and Blood.

Sickness, or states of disease, therefore, are a natural and essential part of life and good health. Seeing illness as a part of our normal state of being may facilitate our "healing" on an emotional, social, spiritual and physical level. The Western view of illness may foster a state of mind that naturally leads to internal conflict and opposition rather than acceptance of illness as a natural aspect of existence and reality.

The philosophical influence of Buddhism in China has also offered a way to explain and understand illness. The Buddha taught that suffering is a result of a deluded mind and one's actions in previous lives, owing to one's karma. (Karma is the idea that we reap what we sow, and is based on the notion that all phenomena are interdependent and arise as an effect and a cause for future conditions.) The spiritual path to alleviate suffering is a gradual process of "seeing reality as it really is." This entails developing self-awareness and insight and shifting one's understanding of reality to the point where the separation between self and other dissolves, and one feels a profound sense of interconnectedness and the arising of deep compassion and acceptance. Illness is not viewed as punishment from a divine creator but as a physical state that can be healed as we realize our attachment to our notion of self and begin to grasp the concept of impermanence. From a Buddhist perspective, there is no "I" that is a fixed composite, a personality, known in my case as Xiaolan. There are only mental and physical processes. It is our holding on to a false sense of "me" that includes "my" body that brings us suffering. Dreading or fearing illness is a manifestation of our attachment to ourselves. By understanding this, we are empowered to move forward and onward from a state of stagnancy and victimization.

It is how we come to understand and give meaning to our illness, such as breast cancer, that brings healing. With cancer, we can still live. There is not an either/or point of view, where we live because we don't have breast cancer and die because we have it. I have met women who have been diagnosed with breast cancer and then have moved into the most rewarding and satisfying phases of their lives. If breast cancer is realized as a spiritual catalyst, then the meaning given it shifts and can be transformed into a process to initiate change and healing.

LAURA

When Laura was forty-seven, she felt a lump in her breast—a growth that hadn't appeared on her last mammogram. She went to see her doctor, who said it was a cyst. Because it seemed to exhibit signs of malignancy, Laura had a fine needle biopsy. The diagnosis was of a pre-cancerous cyst. The doctor told her, "Don't worry about this. Have surgery whenever you can fit it in." Laura decided to go ahead with the surgery. She wasn't worried about it. She had been suffering from ulcerative colitis, a painful bowel disease, for years, and felt that having her cyst removed would be a piece of cake in comparison, like going to the dentist. She told her children about her scheduled surgery the evening before the procedure.

When Laura awoke after the operation, the surgeon was standing over her, looking forlorn. He apologized and told her she had cancer. The cyst had been blocking a tumour, and it wasn't until it was removed that the cancer could be seen. Laura had suffered so much from her bowel disease, that having survived that, she felt she could deal with cancer. The bowel disease was not only extremely painful, but it restricted her greatly. She couldn't leave the house without knowing where the washrooms were located. As well, ulcerative colitis is perceived as a "dirty" disease. She felt awful and found it difficult to feel feminine. She said, "I knew I could get through this breast cancer. It would be such a waste to go through all the suffering around my bowel disease and die." She found strength from past experiences to help her deal with her present challenges.

Laura underwent six months of chemotherapy and six weeks of radiation. She was having a great deal of trouble sleeping and was "living on sleeping pills." She was also experiencing a great deal of pain from her arthritis, which had developed after her bowel disease had escalated. She was prescribed medication for the side effects of chemotherapy, but discovered she was allergic to it when she developed a blood clot.

While Laura was undergoing chemotherapy, she read that women who were in support groups tended to live longer than women going through cancer treatment on their own. She hand-picked seven women to participate in a group. She decided she didn't want a support group with people who were dying, so she would talk to women as they waited to get the results of their blood work. She empowered herself to bring together the support she needed for herself as well as offer it to others.

Laura brought a great deal of humour to the group, as well as to the volunteer work she soon began. She told the women who were undergoing chemo, "Be a princess for six months. Milk it for all it's worth." She wanted to give them hope. She said, "You may think you're supposed to be debilitated, but don't set up your mind to think like this." Laura had a friend who lay drugged on the sofa for six months. She was determined to inform women that it didn't have to be like this. She encouraged women to do what they could to feel as good as they could. She said, "If we look terrible, we feel terrible, and others will feel it too. You'll feel better with some make-up, however much you feel good about putting on."

Laura didn't want to feel like a victim to cancer, so she tried as best she could to live a "normal" life. She scheduled her chemo treatments so she could cook Passover dinner and maintain her family's traditions. She also decided she was going to tell everyone she had cancer. Her experience had been that when people weren't told about an illness, but suspected or heard rumours, they began to imagine the worst-case scenarios and felt uncomfortable. Laura built a strong network of support people who cared about her and who maintained a positive outlook to help her during her challenging and difficult time. Her cancer support group met regularly and, in fact, almost ten years later, is still continuing to meet with some of the original group members.

As Laura went through chemotherapy and radiation, she also started to see me. Her bowel disease was still not under control, even with an artificial bowel. I remember saying to her, "You're dying and it's not the cancer that is killing you. You're not getting enough nutrients to sustain yourself." Laura felt that her doctors were not helping her to any significant degree with her colitis. She would be on intravenous for one month to allow her body to heal, and as soon as she started eating again, she would get sick. Laura was so weak that I started by giving her herbs that are normally prescribed to heal a baby's body. Her health was critically compromised and I wanted to start with something that she could work with. Laura remembers me telling her, "I can help you, but you have to trust me and give yourself time, and you'll have to take an active part in this."

Laura said, "Xiaolan was the first person who understood what I was saying, she wasn't trying to make it better on the surface. She made sense and was very clear in the course of treatment I needed and was very helpful to me, as well as very caring. I trusted her and though the doctors were there, I was reluctant to tell them about the problems that were coming up. I didn't want more medication. It seemed like the only way they could help me was with pills or an operation. In dealing with doctors I felt helpless. In Xiaolan, I found someone who cared enough to help me find the key."

Laura went on a diet that consisted of more fresh produce and fish, and less meat. She began to eat tofu and started listening to her body. Over time, she was able to eat without becoming ill. She was also able to stop taking medication for her migraines, which had been so severe that she had sometimes gone to the hospital for Demerol shots. As she regained her strength she was able to achieve healing at a deep level.

Laura has courageously gone through so many difficulties in her life, but says, "I think breast cancer was the best thing to happen. Maybe it gave me the push to really live." She was able to trust in her ability to work with her breast cancer and her bowel disease to pursue new meaning in her life. She firmly believes that it is our mindset and attitudes that really make the difference in our ability to heal, as well as the supportive, caring relationships we form with ourselves and with others.

Relationships that allow and facilitate our growth into wholeness are critical when we are ill. We each need to share our ups and downs with another who cares and understands. It is not the number of relationships that matter, but the quality. Without close relationships we may feel ignored and depressed, with feelings of emptiness and isolation. Healing relationships provide us with opportunities to share and not be judged. They satisfy our need to feel the empathy of another. Someone enters our world as though it were their own, and the intimacy and caring that this type of relationship engenders is a significant factor in surviving disease.

SUPPORT AFTER CANCER TREATMENT

Chemotherapy drugs and radiation tend to deplete the Spleen and weaken Kidney Essence, or Jing. Drug therapy harms the Stomach lining and Intestines, resulting in nausea, vomiting and loss of appetite and absorption of nutrients. Spleen Qi, which is critical to the transformation and transportation of Blood, is also damaged. Therefore any self-care we can undertake to support our Spleen is beneficial after chemotherapy.

DIET

The following foods weaken the Spleen and should be avoided after cancer treatment:

- cold, frozen and raw foods
- dairy products
- rich, greasy foods
- strongly spiced foods
- sweets

In addition, we should not consume stimulating foods and drinks such as chocolate, caffeine and alcohol since they can disrupt the flow of Liver Qi. We should eat moderate amounts at regular times. Eating too little or too much food can harm the body.

PHYSICAL EXERCISE

Balanced physical exertion helps support the Spleen. We should try to maintain an appropriate balance between rest and work; neither too much rest nor overwork are supportive of the body.

ACUPRESSURE

Self-care acupressure as described on pages 96 to 98, can activate the flow of Qi and enhance the Spleen and Kidney networks.

QI GONG

Qi Gong nourishes and supports the Spleen, Liver and Kidneys, which are weakened during cancer treatment. Cancer patients are often encouraged to practise this ancient Chinese art.

KIM

Sixteen years ago a cancer diagnosis was a total shock to Kim. She was a physical education teacher and counsellor, was very fit and lived on a macrobiotic diet. She underwent a modified radical mastectomy, which removes the entire breast and axillary lymph nodes in the underarm area. Kim knew she needed to learn to live with her breast cancer, so she decided to attend a class offered through the local cancer centre, even though she is not a group person. She participated in the "Healing Journey" classes at Princess Margaret Hospital in Toronto, where she learned skills such as relaxation, meditation and visualization. This was a fairly big stretch for her. Meditation was pretty "weird" in her mind, but she was willing to try.

These classes were transformational for Kim. She was able to learn spiritual and psychological ways of coping with breast cancer, while being treated with the drug Tamoxifen. In these classes, Kim began a profound spiritual journey, questioning who she was and what was important to her. She learned relaxation techniques in the meditation and visualization classes, and also had the opportunity to express her deep feelings and learn new ways to be with them and deal with them effectively. Two years later, she went for a checkup and was given a clean bill of health. She was ecstatic and celebrated by taking a bottle of wine to her doctor.

Less than one month later, as she was driving, she noticed her hands were puffy. Within two months the swelling progressively worsened until her entire shoulder area was black and swollen. Her breast cancer had spread to underneath her collarbone, where it was pinching nerves and blood vessels. Kim was told that this was an extremely difficult area to treat. Even if she had her arm and shoulder amputated, the cancer would not stop growing. She was directed to one of the best radiation oncologists in Canada, who told her that he could provide relief of her symptoms but that she should consider the radiation palliative, and not a cure.

Kim continued her meditation and visualization and heard about various places to go for healing. She didn't know what to do or where to go. At one of her meditation seminars, she asked the facilitator where she should go for healing. The facilitator said, "If there is healing anywhere in the world, it can be found right here." This was what Kim needed to hear. When she'd first been diagnosed with breast cancer, she had tried to do everything possible and perfectly to recover, and yet her cancer returned. She began to question the nature of healing. Was healing already present within her? How could she access it?

Kim tried yoga but found that she couldn't do the exercises because of her shoulder. She then decided to try Qi Gong, which was being offered at a local cancer support centre. Qi

Gong happened to align with her beliefs about healing, which were that self-healing is possible and has happened through-out history. The concept of tapping into healing energy to bring harmony and balance to her body resonated strongly with her. In fact, she likens healing to a thread that connects all of existence and believes that it is up to each of us to do our best to tap into this energy.

One year after the reoccurrence of her cancer, Kim embraced the practice of Qi Gong. To the astonishment of her doctors, Kim was alive the following year, and her tumour had disappeared. She has continued her Qi Gong practice and now teaches classes herself. She works on developing com-passion for her body, healing emotionally, mentally, physically and spiritually, and allowing the healing energy to move through her.

Kim is very careful about talking about "cures." For her, living in the present moment without cancer is where she is on her healing journey. Unsure of what tomorrow may hold, Kim says, "Life is a mystery . . . let it unfold."

Here are the Qi Gong exercises that Kim practises daily:

THE HORSE

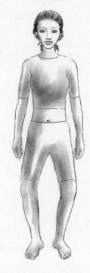 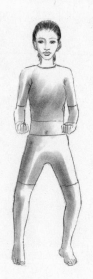 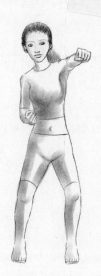

Stand with feet together, arms at sides of the body. Weight is forward on the feet. Back is straight. When breathing in, inhale through the soles of the feet to the *Dan Tian*, a point below the naval, and into the Lungs. Take a few deep breaths. Step out to the left, a distance that feels comfortable. Keep knees soft and slightly bent. Slowly bring hands held in a fist to rest on the top of the hips. Palms of the hands should be facing up. Punch out first with the right arm. Breathe out with the forward movement of the arm. Many of us find that exaggerating our out-breath, combined with the punching motion, is a wonderful way to express and release pent-up frustration and anger. Return the hand to rest on the top of the hip. Repeat with left arm. Begin with three punches per arm, then increase to five, then to seven. Return arms to the sides of the body. Straighten knees. Bring left leg beside the right.

POINTING TO THE MOON

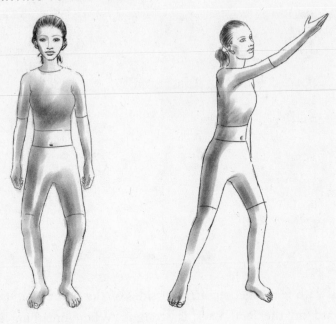

This exercise is very beneficial for lymphedema, a condition where swelling occurs as lymph fluid pools in the tissues of the arms and legs. This condition may develop after breast surgery or radiation therapy. Breathe from the soles of the feet to the *Dan Tian*, a point below the naval, and into the Lungs. Weight is forward on feet. Back is straight. Keep knees soft and slightly bent. Stand or sit, arms at sides. If standing, step out to the left, a distance that feels comfortable. Pinch the thumb and the third finger together on each hand. Hold hands with palms facing up beside the body. Beginning with right arm, while breathing out, swing up from beside the body, diagonally across the chest to a point as high above the left side of the body as is comfortable. Follow your fingers with your eyes. Then drop and swing up with the left arm. A natural swinging rhythm will develop. Remember to breathe out with each upward swing. Begin with three swings per side, then increase to five, then to seven. Return arms to the side of the body. Straighten knees. Bring left leg beside the right.

THE CRANE

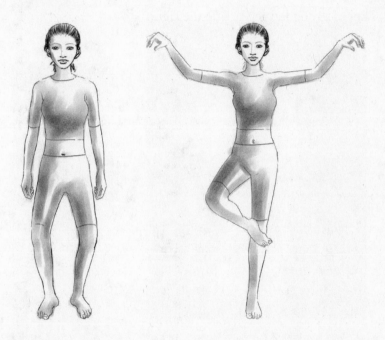

This is a revealing exercise as it tends to tell us if our minds are elsewhere while we are practising. It requires concentration and focus that is more difficult if we're thinking of what to make for dinner, or how we're going to accomplish everything on our to-do list. Check posture and breathing. Keep arms, shoulders and wrists soft. Step out to the left. Focus on a spot on the floor or the wall. Breathing in, transfer weight to one foot, whichever one feels most natural. Raise the unweighted foot and place beside or behind the knee, breathing in. Slowly raise arms out, palms up to the sides to shoulder height. Hold pose and hold breath. Then, while breathing out, slowly lower foot to floor, and lower arms to the sides. Now shift weight to other foot and repeat. Try to keep all movements slow and smooth. Return arms to the sides of the body. Straighten knees. Bring left leg beside the right.

THE BEAR

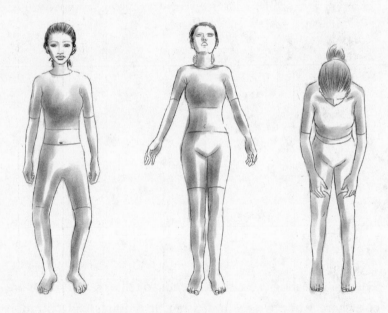

Step out to the left, a distance that feels comfortable. Keep knees soft and slightly bent. Keep entire body loose and soft. Breathing out, arch back, move head and shoulders back as far as it feels comfortable. Move arms up slightly, with palms open upwards; this is very good for opening up the chest. Then, breathing out, collapse forward, knees soft, shoulders rounded, driving air out of our lungs, letting go. Slowly repeat. Return arms to the sides of the body. Straighten knees. Bring left leg beside the right.

HEALING AND CURING

I believe that people have the ability to self-heal and that once they understand their capacity to do so, they will move to fulfill their potential for wellness. I think it's important to distinguish healing from curing. I see healing as the process of becoming whole and finding meaning in our circumstances. It involves harmonizing all aspects of ourselves—physical, emotional, mental and spiritual. The Chinese word that refers to all these levels is *xin*, meaning "heart-mind." Figure 7 shows the Chinese character for *xin*.

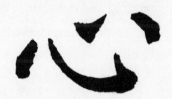

Figure 7: Xin

Curing is generally focused on eliminating or reducing symptoms or disease. It usually involves working with the body or a body process. Treatment is focused on stopping, controlling or removing a specific condition. Generally, the responsibility of curing is given to another, usually a health-care practitioner. Healing is something we direct ourselves. When we understand what it is to heal, we know that a specific physical or physiological condition does not have to restrict the quality of our life. Our lives encompass more than the material, our physicality. Healing helps us to connect to who we are within a "larger" context, whatever we understand this to be. It brings our inner sense of solitariness into relationship with something "greater" than ourselves. We are in synch, in harmony, with ourselves and our environments. Even if curing is not possible, healing can still occur.

All this is not to say that healing and curing are two distinct approaches to disease; both are needed. Trained in Western medicine, I recognize the need to deal with acute, physical symptoms that are painful and debilitating. As a TCM practitioner I also understand the importance of finding and working with the root causes of disease and distress. Health is not merely the absence of disease, it's about living in harmony will all levels of ourselves, *xin*, and recognizing that this is a changing and dynamic state of being.

SUMMARY

Breast disorders represent a continuum of conditions that follow a progression. Symptoms that are often considered normal accompaniments to the flow of Heavenly Water, such as breast distension and tenderness, indicate imbalances within the Organ systems and, if left untreated, can intensify over time and accumulate to increasingly more serious and deepseated disorders. The conditions in the continuum are fed by the same underlying causes, and indicate an evolution of disorder over a prolonged period of time. At the extreme end of the continuum is *Ru Yan,* or breast cancer.

The root cause of breast conditions is most often emotional disturbances such as anger, frustration, unfulfilled desires and overthinking. When these emotions do not move smoothly, as when we repress or explosively vent them, or let them continue to cycle through our minds, over time they will adversely affect the free flow of Qi in the breasts. To maintain breast health, it is vital that we learn to manage and reduce emotional stress in a healthy way. Learning how to positively deal with emotional stress will go a tremendous distance in caring for our breasts and preventing illness.

As well, we should maintain a proper diet, be moderate in physical and mental exertion and be mindful of the general risk factors that make us more susceptible to breast disorders. We can also support Qi and deal with our emotions and stress through the practice of restorative exercises such as Qi Gong.

To heal is to bring harmony to the Three Treasures—the physical, the emotional and the spiritual. Healing from a disease such as breast cancer is a journey towards wholeness, which embraces the integration and balance of the different manifestations of Qi, that is, Jing, Qi and Shen—the harmonious working together of our body, mind and spirit.

Part Four

CLOUDS AND RAIN

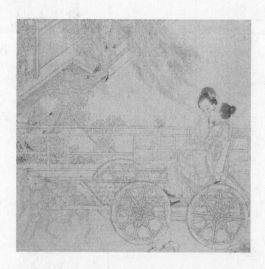

Amorous couple, ink on silk, by Jiao Bingzhen
(1622–1723 AD)

CHAPTER NINE

Sex and Well-Being

*I*n Traditional Chinese Medicine, sex is an important factor in maintaining good health—as important as food and sleep. Not only is sex a tremendous source of pleasure and fulfillment, but it is a means to attain increased energy, physical well-being and a long lifespan, as well as an expression of our wholeness as a human being.

The ancient Taoists described sexual intercourse metaphorically as *yun-yu*, or "clouds and rain." For them, clouds represented the woman's essence, her vaginal secretions, while rain referred to the emission of semen. Their use of natural allusions to describe sex illustrates that they regarded it as a natural and necessary part of life. Unlike in the West, where sex was more often than not historically imbued with guilt and identified as either good in the context of marriage or reprehensible outside of it, the ancient Chinese did not form moral judgments about sex. Instead, they saw it as the natural interplay between Yin and Yang. Since ancient practitioners sought to achieve health and longevity through a balance between Yin and Yang, sexual relations were explored as a means to enhance one's health.

When sex is engaged in, bodily fluids intermingle and breathing synchronizes so that neither Yin nor Yang dominates the other. The hot, fiery, short-lived Yang energy is balanced with cool, enduring Yin energy. Sexual intercourse with orgasm helps women nurture their Yin energy by absorbing Yang, while men absorb Yin to support their Yang. Sex is the harmonizing of water and fire. As fire is required to heat and boil water, men must excite women with their fire, or Yang energy. Once the fiery energy is exhausted, ashes are all that remain. But water will remain warm for a period of time, even after the fire has gone out. Men's fire is quick to start and quick to die out, while women's water takes time to boil and time to cool down. This is interpreted to mean that women have the capability to experience limitless orgasms, whereas a man is prone to sleep after sex, sapped of his energy upon ejaculation.

The ancient Taoists believed that a man's semen was his Essence, or Jing. Frequent ejaculation, then, could deplete his vital Essence, accelerate the aging process, and result in ill health and a shortened life. Men were advised to engage in regular sex but to ejaculate for procreation only in order to preserve their Essence. This did not mean that they weren't supposed to orgasm every time they had sex. According to the Taoists, ejaculation and orgasm were not one and the same event. Because they occur in quick succession, it is usually assumed they are indistinguishable. However, ejaculation, as a physical release of seminal fluid from the body, is separate from climax, which is a pleasurable, intense feeling that can be experienced throughout the entire body. To stop semen from being discharged, one recommended technique was to apply pressure to the perineum, a point located between the anus and scrotum prior to and during orgasm. Men also learned breathing exercises as another means to prevent ejaculation.

This Taoist teaching of controlling the discharge of semen has been countered by some in Western medicine who hold that when ejaculation occurs, the prostate gland swells with stimulation and then contracts. With the absence of ejaculation, there is no contraction and a risk that the prostate could become enlarged. The glands that secrete the seminal fluid may cease to function properly and eventually weaken, decreasing sexual capability and the capacity to ejaculate. The Taoists, however, believed that the retention of seminal fluid would increase a man's sexual capacity by fortifying his vitality. Additionally, by controlling the discharge of semen, a man would be able to participate in sexual intercourse until his partner achieved orgasm, at which time he was able to absorb her Yin energy.

Though the Taoist teachings on sex were directed towards men, there was also the recognition that both sexes needed to reach orgasm. As complementary opposites, both Yin and Yang had to be stimulated and aroused for perfect union. Though women discharge fluids when they orgasm, these secretions are held within their body, so women are not at the same risk as men of losing their vitality. Women retain their Essence and are able to absorb Yang energy to strengthen them. In this way women were considered stronger, with a larger capacity for sex, greater sexual hunger and more sexual energy. Water is stronger than fire—it can, after all, put a fire out.

Reciprocal gathering of the other sex's secretions was considered by the ancients as important to balance the Yin and Yang energies in men and women. However, it should be noted that within each female there is both Yin and Yang energy, as there is both Yang and Yin energy within males. In some instances, women may have a predominance of Yang energy, while some men may have an abundance of Yin energy. A female with strong internal Yang energy can be balanced through absorbing Yin during sex with another female. Since women have unlimited resources of Yin energy, and there is no loss of Yin during sex, lesbianism would not be considered detrimental to health or affect one's lifespan. In the same way, a male who is mostly Yin can absorb Yang Essence from another male. However, if the men are not well versed in the art of retaining semen, sexual relations could result in a depletion of Yang energy and Essence for both.

For the Taoists, then, sexual intercourse was not about releasing energies and emotions, but rather the opposite: a means to replenish sexual energy and ensure physical, emotional and mental well-being. They also believed that sex could be a spiritual experience, since it was a bringing together of complementary opposites to unite with the macrocosm of heaven and earth. Depletion of sexual energy was said to result in an emptiness of the mind and senses. When this occurs, we may repress our sexual needs or search for fulfillment of our desires by looking for other sources of stimulation, such as alcohol or drugs, in an attempt to build up the much needed internal energy that we've exhausted. However in partaking of liquor or narcotics, we end up further depleting our energy. We may become obsessive in our quest for greater stimulation to make up for the energy drained from us. A vicious cycle is underway, as our energy is consumed, our mind and body become further weakened, resulting in an increased desire for enhanced stimulation, which only serves to further impoverish us energetically. Our senses become over-activated and our Essence dwindles away.

So it is important that we not suppress our sexual energy, disregard it, nor allow it to run out of control. Frequent sexual intercourse with orgasms is one of the most effective means for women to nurture their sexual energy and Essence.

CHAPTER TEN

Women's Experiences of Sex

Though a satisfying sex life will contribute greatly to a woman's overall health and well-being, many of us may not, unfortunately, have harmonious and complementary sex lives. We may not experience sex as a creative energy that stimulates our passion, nourishes our inner world, or fortifies our internal energy. Many women are dissatisfied with their sexual experiences, and there are a number of factors—internal and external—that contribute to this discontent, the foremost two perhaps being cultural and societal forces.

Growing up in China, I was never told with words, but somehow I just knew not to talk to the boy who sat next to me in primary school. I envisioned an imaginary line that separated his space from mine, a boundary that we both silently acknowledged would not be crossed. I didn't make eye contact with him, let alone talk to or touch him. I was incredibly fearful of the consequences that would result if I interacted verbally or physically with a member of the opposite sex. As I reflect back, it has been difficult to articulate exactly what it was that I feared. It wasn't as if my mother told me I would be reprimanded by her, or that the teacher would object. No, it was a tacit understanding among everyone, parents, teachers, us children, that boys and girls who engaged in personal conversation, such as "How are you?" or "Have you eaten?" or who touched, would be ostracized, ridiculed and shamed for being "bad." A simple interaction between a boy and girl became connected with sin, filth, disgrace and degradation, which would dishonour my family and prove I was not a worthy daughter.

As I grew older, this anxiety escalated. As teens and young adults, my generation was terrified to even feel the emotions that were beginning to stir for members of the opposite sex. I remember struggling not to think of young men in a romantic way. When I was in high school, there was a male student whom I was drawn to. I admired his mind and on several occasions found my gaze focused on him. Soon I heard whispers behind my back: "Xiaolan likes Y"; "Did you see her looking at him?"; "What are they doing?" The rumours were starting based on my innocent looks of admiration. I was terrified others would know I was attracted to this young man and would ostracize me in a society where conformity was paramount.

This was how it was in China in the seventies, a time when Communism ruled and the impact of Confucian thought still prevailed. Confucius taught an ethical way for everyone to conduct themselves in society, with specific obligations required of each relationship, be it spouses, parents and children, ruler and subjects, that if adhered to, would result in a righteous and harmonious society. Women were designated with a role that equated their value with their dutifulness to husbands, fathers and sons. Additionally, Confucianism, being very pragmatic, considered sex's primary purpose as procreation, more specifically, to produce sons. Romantic love and passion were denigrated since they would separate a son from his bond with his parents, thereby upsetting the hierarchy of the family structure.

The arrival of Communism only deepened this repressive attitude to sex. Although the Communists opposed the strict Confucian gender roles and established the equality of women as a significant aspect of reform, they viewed passionate desire and love as possible threats to political and social stability. We were told that romantic love and sex were indulgences of the bourgeois class, whose focus was personal desire and therefore damaging to collective well-being. We were to express our passion for the revolution and not our "weaknesses" by falling in love. Manifestations of sexuality were suppressed; public displays of affection, even holding hands, were unacceptable.

Growing up in such a milieu as this, it is not surprising that my husband and I entered marriage with no understanding of sex. I fumbled through the mechanics of it with no awareness that it could be a highly pleasurable experience. The majority of my friends shared my ignorance, and I later discovered that our husbands generally devoted less than a minute to foreplay and were focused on satisfying themselves with no thought of enjoyment for us women. And, we women didn't question what was happening in our bedrooms. We accepted our lot. We focused on ensuring that we fulfilled our duties as good wives, that is, ensuring our husbands were satisfied, so they wouldn't go outside the marriage to have sex, as well as continuing the family with the birth of a son.

After I'd been running my clinic in Canada for a number of years, I came to realize that many Western women feel a similar distaste of, or lack of enjoyment of, sex. I can remember the day Anne, a patient I had been working with for a few years, told me, "I don't enjoy sex, and it's come to the point where I'd rather my husband satisfy his sexual needs elsewhere, rather than me doing something that I so dislike." When I heard these words, I felt honoured, surprised and confused simultaneously. I felt honoured that Anne would share these confidential thoughts with me, and surprised that Anne would sanction and perhaps even encourage her husband to seek sex outside the marriage. I was also surprised that she, as a Western woman who had come through the sexual revolution and freedom of the sixties, would feel as disinterested in sex as Chinese women of my generation.

Since then, a large number of my patients have confided in me about their dissatisfaction with their sex lives. Some women feel they don't do it "right"; others are bored with it and see it as another item on their chore list. For some, sexual intercourse feels uncomfortable or painful; while others feel they aren't desirable. There are even those who feel something is wrong with their sexuality because they have no desire or can't achieve orgasm. Since the fifties, women have become more visible in the workplace than ever before; laws have been passed stipulating equal pay for equal work and prohibiting discrimination on the basis of sex or marital status; women have more control over their fertility; sex and women's sexuality are more openly discussed in the media; there are more manuals, guides and therapists to enhance our sex lives, to name just a few of the significant gains, but many women's sexual experiences haven't really changed. Perhaps this is because the sexual revolution did not necessarily lead to equality in the area of sexual satisfaction.

While men have celebrated their sexuality, women who do so may still be branded as a "whore" or a "tramp," with an accompanying fall in self-esteem, social acceptance and financial stability. Women have been taught to believe that men seek partners who are chaste and morally virtuous. If we subscribe to this morality, we may suppress our own sexual impulses. In this way, we cede our sexual independence for social acceptance and desirability as a partner.

As well, we are inundated in this society with images of idealized female bodies in advertisements, magazines and movies that tell us what "attractive" and "sexy" look like. If we don't fit the idealized standard, if we are too heavy or flat-chested or not pretty enough or too old, we may not see ourselves as attractive and sexy. Finding ourselves lacking, we develop negative body images, and our self-esteem plummets. The perception we have of ourselves and our personal worth is an important factor in sexual satisfaction. Women need to feel valued and respected during sex, not self-conscious or criticized. Our concentration on appearances and our negative body images hinder us from fully engaging in sexual relations, leaving us feeling inadequate, undesirable and unenthusiastic about sex.

This brings to mind a story about frogs that I once heard. A group of frogs were hopping through the woods, and two of them fell into a very deep hole. All the other frogs gathered around the edge of the hole and looked down. "Friends," they yelled, "the hole is very deep, we're not sure how you will be able to get out." The two frogs began jumping with all of their might, trying to get out of the hole. The other frogs at the top of the hole said, "Oh my goodness, it's too deep! You should stop trying; it's too far to the top!" The two frogs kept trying and hit themselves against the side of the hole in their attempts. The frogs at the edge of the hole could hardly bear to watch. They shouted, "Please stop, you're hurting your-selves, it's no use!" Finally one of the frogs took heed of what the others were saying and gave up. It sat down and became despondent and depressed. But the other frog continued to jump as hard as it could until it made a huge leap and got out! The other frogs gathered round and asked, "Didn't you hear us telling you to stop?" The frog said, "I'm hard of hearing. I thought you were cheering me on."

This story is about the power of words and messages. The one frog, believing he was being encouraged by the others, was able to overcome seemingly insurmountable obstacles. The same message was given to both frogs, but it was the belief inside each of them that seemed to make the difference in how they were equipped to deal with the situation. Analogously, we women all hear similar messages about what we should look like and wear to be valued, but isn't it what we do with these messages that makes the difference? Can we form our own beliefs about the value of who are, so we aren't so reliant on what others say? Can we hold on to these beliefs and not allow others' words and messages to affect us?

I think of how often the voices that we need to be deaf to are not only external voices, but also our own internal voices that tell us, "My body isn't in shape so why would my partner want me?" or "I'm too old to be thinking of sex." We can listen to these voices and feel undesirable, inadequate or at fault, or we can choose to be deaf to these voices and offer words of encouragement to ourselves. We can start to believe in ourselves as sexual beings, unique and beautiful in our own way. And, perhaps, in so doing, we can begin to trust in our sexuality and explore what we desire and enjoy, allowing our sexual energy to flow unimpeded.

Judging by the type of advertising and magazine articles we see, one might think a woman's raison d'être was to fulfill a man's desires and wants. It seems women are conditioned to accept stereotypes of women and men that reinforce notions of what we must look like and do to keep men happy. When the emphasis in sex is on men's desires and satisfaction, there is less room for the fulfillment of our own needs. Women fake orgasms because we want to please our partners. We are concerned that our partners may feel inadequate if we don't climax, since we've been told that so much of men's self-esteem is connected to their sexual prowess, and to threaten our partner's self-esteem may endanger the very foundation of our relationship. We feel it is easier to fake an orgasm then achieve a real one and we don't want our partners to feel obligated to keep trying. Orgasms are beyond the realm of possibility for us so it's better to get sex over with. We fake them and tell ourselves it's not as important for us as it is for a man to climax. So much of why we lie about achieving orgasms is based on promoting our partner's feeling of sexual well-being. Why are we so concerned about how our partners are feeling at the expense of our needs and desires?

EXPLORING OUR SEXUAL IDENTITY

It seems that we have lost touch with who we are sexually and what we want. Somehow we must try to go beyond the social, cultural and personal factors that predispose us towards forgoing our own needs. I feel that realizing we may not be connected to our own desires is a key to understanding and transforming our sex lives. We need to re-examine our beliefs and feelings in order to cultivate our sexual potential. I feel strongly that one of the most important beliefs for us to embrace is that women deserve and are entitled to sexual satisfaction and enjoyment. And we deserve this without first fulfilling our partners' needs. We have the right to fully feel our own sexual desires and feelings, whatever they may be, and then have them met. And, of course this means getting in touch with what it is we truly want sexually. If we do not know what we desire, what arouses us, what feels good or not, how can we know ourselves as sexual beings? Men don't give us orgasms, it is we who facilitate our own. This is an empowering idea, because it is we who determine our sexual satisfaction. We are not helpless victims but active participants.

How do we feel about ourselves when we connect to our own sexuality? To honestly be in touch with a deep and intimate aspect of ourselves allows us to know ourselves better, and accept and value who we are. Again we must ignore the discouraging internal voices that might say, "Sex isn't a pleasurable experience" or "I'm so ridiculous that I feel some fear in exploring my sexuality" or "I just can't speak to a man about what I desire sexually." Instead we must encourage ourselves with supportive words and actions. When we become in synch with ourselves, we may find our emotions are less deadened or less volatile. When we have satisfying sex lives, we may find that we sleep better, that our eating habits are no longer out of control and that we have more energy. All of these factors contribute significantly to our overall health, including our emotional health. If we are not happy with our sexual lives, our emotions will detrimentally impact our bodies, minds and spirit.

RACHEL

Rachel is a very successful woman with whom men are quickly enchanted. When she became serious with one man, she was afflicted with a series of recurring urinary tract infections. After several bouts, she came to see me. As we talked, I asked her about her relationship. Rachel told me that her boyfriend "wanted sex all the time," but because of her infections, she wasn't interested in sex. The more we talked, Rachel explained that she felt her boyfriend was with her primarily for sex. On one level, she was hurt by him because she felt he wasn't genuinely interested in what she had to say or what she was excited about. As the relationship progressed, the frequency of the infections increased. I asked Rachel if she felt that her urinary tract infections could be a way for her to avoid sex with her boyfriend or to "get back" at him for the hurt she felt. As Rachel had begun to feel that her worth to her boyfriend was connected to her sexual willingness and attractiveness, she had felt not only hurt but angry as well. She felt that all of her wasn't being valued, and she began to resent her boyfriend.

Shortly after our discussion, Rachel decided to break off the relationship. And, over the next while, her urinary tract infections subsided. She subsequently entered into another relationship with a man who supported and encouraged her. When she last came to see me, she hadn't had an infection for over two years. Rachel was able to connect with her feelings of hurt and anger and then make a different choice that valued her. And, in so doing, her urinary tract infections stopped and she enjoyed regular sexual activity.

In sexual relations, which are so intimate, there are many opportunities for us to feel accepted or rejected. How we feel about our sexuality has far-reaching implications outside of the bedroom, influencing how we feel about ourselves overall, which we express through our emotions, words, thoughts and actions. When we have a satisfying sex life, we have more confidence in who we are, our worth and what we bring to a relationship. If we feel we have intrinsic value in who we are, we will not be at the mercy of the messages put forth by others. We may find that we make choices so we don't neglect ourselves. We take care of ourselves in a loving and compassionate way that supports our bodies, hearts and minds. We don't feel the need to put our partners' sexual satisfaction ahead of our own because we become an integral part of the sexual equation. We have value and are equally entitled to sexual fulfillment, because we now value ourselves.

Okay, you may be thinking, I cognitively accept that this is all true, but how do I get in touch with what I desire sexually? The answer to this question will differ for each of us, depending on our histories, the society we've grown up in and the primary influences in our lives. In my case, I've had to explore how I feel about sex and about myself as a sexual being. What does sexual attraction mean to me and how do I feel physically and emotionally when I am attracted to another? How do I enjoy my body, what is it that arouses me? What satisfies me sexually? I admit that when I first started exploring these questions, I felt overwhelmed and at a loss as to how to even begin to understand what the questions meant to me, never mind trying to tackle answering them. Perhaps you too may find yourselves feeling this way. If so, then I would like to share what helped me.

First, I needed to take the time to discover what it is that I feel about sex. I began with the intention of exploring this. Continual sincere intention has the power to activate action, for without intention, activity, thoughts and words will never arise. If we consciously, and with honest intent, desire to explore our sexuality, we will find ourselves setting aside time. It's also important to feel what happens in our bodies as we take the time to explore our sexuality and ask ourselves questions about how we feel. When I thought, talked about, wrote about or watched a movie about sex, I checked in to see what was going on in my body. I paid attention to the feelings, the subtle shifts, the tingling sensations, the heaviness, the fluttering, etc. I determined whether I was feeling afraid, excited or angry.

Connecting with our bodies and opening to them fully and consciously is so necessary if we want to know what it is that we desire and like. If you do so, try to withhold judgment about what is "right" or "wrong," as well as preconceptions of what arises, be it a feeling, sensation, thought, like or dislike. Many of us will confront our sexual desires or erotic impulses with moral judgment before we even have a chance to know how we fully feel, before we connect with the intensity of them, or before we've formed a sense of whether this is something we actually like or want, or just something we feel we are expected to want. Observe any feelings of shame, embarrassment or guilt for feeling attracted to a person or to an action or a situation that takes you off guard and goes beyond your comfort zone. We may find ourselves going headfirst into some of our strongest emotions when we explore our desires, and into censure when we connect with our feelings. Try to be patient and to be with the feelings, sensations and thoughts long enough to identify them: "This feels good"; "I am feeling hurt"; "I am feeling excited"; "I am afraid"; "I like this"; "I feel guilty"; "I am uncomfortable." Connecting to what we feel about sex, a person, an act, or ourselves as sexual beings is critical to learning to accept and feel good about our bodies, the way we feel, smell, move or look dressed or undressed. Understanding what we want and desire sexually will help us make positive changes in our sex lives and ultimately in our relationships with ourselves as well as with others.

Keep in mind that how we feel sexually will change and evolve over time. How I felt about sex twenty years ago is radically different than how I feel about it today, and I have no doubt my feelings will continue to change as I age. For example, a person whom I was sexually attracted to several years ago may no longer hold the same attraction for me. But in spite of all the changes that happen, the constant is my connection with what I feel about myself as a sexual being. I have a sense of who I am and have the confidence to know what *I* desire.

Once we have connected to ourselves as sexual beings, Taoism teaches many practices to promote sexual energy. These include physical movement, breathing exercises, massage, visualizations, meditations and sexual techniques to balance our Yin and Yang so as to reap the benefits of sexual intercourse.* One method of cultivating sexual energy is through the Microcosmic Orbit.

THE MICROCOSMIC ORBIT

During this breathing and visualization technique, sexual energy is drawn up the Governing Vessel, or Yang Channel that starts at the perineum, which is between the vagina and the anus, then travels up the spine, around the head, then down towards the roof of the mouth. Touching the tongue to the palate behind the front teeth closes the circuit by connecting the Conception Vessel or Yin Channel, which begins at the perineum, then runs up the front of the torso, over the pubic bone, through the internal organs, up the throat, terminating at the end of the tongue (see Figure 8).

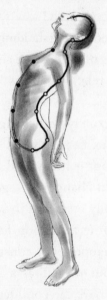

To become aware of the Microcosmic Orbit, we need to take a few minutes to sit quietly and focus inward. Find a place and a time where you will not be interrupted and sit, stand or lie comfortably. Allow your body and breathing to relax. Place your

Figure 8: The Microcosmic Orbit

---

* "These practices are described in the ancient texts *The Handbook of the Plain Girl* and *The Art of the Bedchamber.*

hands on your abdomen, with your thumbs in the area of your navel and your index fingers joined—this creates a kind of triangle over the ovaries, where female sexual energy is stored. Place your tongue against the roof of your mouth, behind the front teeth. Inhaling through your nose, focus on the area under your hands.

At first, there may not be anything that we feel. Or we may become aware of a feeling of warmth, of subtle energy. This energy begins in the area of the navel, and travels first down to the perineum. This is an important point in Chinese medicine—it is the seat of Jing energy. The energy then flows up the spine, up over the back of the head, down the front of the face to the roof of the mouth, through the tongue, down the throat, the front of the torso, over the pubic bone, back to the perineum, then circulates through the loop again. Try to feel the energy moving by focusing on where it is travelling through the circuit. With practice, we will feel it circling down the front and then back up the body. There may be tingling or a feeling of arousal. Try taking time each day to practise this simple yet highly effective and powerful meditation, which enhances sexual pleasure and circulates energy to the various parts of the body, bringing balance and healing as well as slowing the process of aging.

SUMMARY

In Traditional Chinese Medicine, satisfying sex is considered necessary for good health and longevity. This perspective can be traced back to the ancient Taoists who viewed life as a dynamic interplay of complementary opposites, of which women, Yin, and men, Yang, are but one manifestation. The bringing together of Yin and Yang has spiritual and emotional benefits, which will be embodied in physical well-being and harmonious relationships with ourselves and others.

Chinese women of my generation understand the role that sex plays in health, but our attitudes towards sex have been radically influenced by Confucianism and Communism. Both of these belief systems are based on the understanding that sex and passion have the power to divide family members or to separate one's loyalty from the Party, and thus held that sex was detrimental to the family unit and society.

Sex for many women, Chinese as well as Western, isn't enjoyable or satisfying. Though the reasons for this dissatisfaction are varied, one explanation stands above the others: we focus on our partners' satisfaction over what we need and desire.

In the West, women have been sexually objectified, but in some ways we are complicit in perpetuating this view. We continue to equate our value with how we look, how well we meet the culturally constructed ideal of the desirable, sexy woman. In focusing on male satisfaction and ignoring our own, we have lost our identities and subscribed to how men may define us. But our sexual satisfaction is no less important than men's. In fact the ancient Taoists believed that women are sexually more powerful than men. Both Yin and Yang must be stimulated and satisfied for balance, and sexual energy helps us achieve physical, emotional and mental health, vigour and an increased lifespan. With these benefits, it is not just that women have the right to a satisfying sex life, it is something we should actively pursue. It is my wholehearted wish that we may realize and experience the vitality and physical health that accompanies owning our sexual energy, which is an integral aspect of who we are as healthy, confident women.

Part Five

RIPENING THE FRUIT

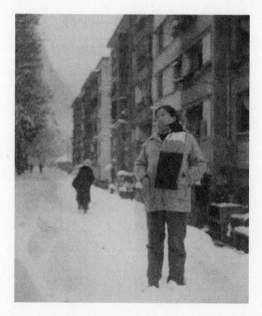

Me, pregnant with my son, Zhao Zhao,
in January 1984

CHAPTER ELEVEN

Planting the Seed

In Traditional Chinese Medicine, the Kidney system is responsible for human reproduction, growth and development. The Kidneys are where we store our Jing, or Essence, which is the foundation of the body and its functions, and can be transformed into Qi. There are two kinds of Essence. The first is prenatal Essence, which is the genetic material we inherit from our parents when we are conceived. It endows us with our unique constitution, vitality and nature. We each have a finite amount of prenatal Essence and use a little each day to produce and move the Qi in our bodies. Once we've depleted it, as we do through the course of our lives, we naturally die. The second type of Essence is postnatal Essence, which we produce from the food we eat and how we live our lives. If we have abundant postnatal Essence, we use up less of our prenatal Essence, and thereby prolong our life.

The strength of our Essence, or Kidney Qi, is also a significant factor in conception and determines the health and vitality of our children. The parents' Essence forms their babies' prenatal Essence, which sustains and nourishes them in the womb and throughout their lives. Therefore, both parents' constitutional health, age and state of well-being at conception all contribute to their babies' health. If the parents' Kidneys are weakened due to a constitutional deficiency, aging or overwork, this may result in inadequate Essence, which may lead to possible problems in conceiving, and infertility and, if conception has occurred, lack of nourishment for the fetus to properly develop and grow.

If we plan to have children, then, it is important that we try to support our Kidney Essence. We can endeavour to preserve our prenatal Essence by avoiding overwork and excessive physical exertion (this includes strenuous activities such as sports), irregular dietary habits, inadequate rest and chronic illness. We may also support our prenatal Essence by increasing our postnatal Essence. The food and drinks we consume are manufactured into Blood and Qi and used for our daily activities. At the end of the day, if there is surplus Blood and Qi, it will be transformed into postnatal Essence and stored in our Kidneys. To support the manufacture of abundant postnatal Essence, we can do our best to maintain a proper diet, stay away from exposure to Cold and Damp conditions, deal with our stress and emotions appropriately, abstain from or reduce our consumption of coffee, tobacco and alcohol, and maintain regular work and rest patterns. A proper diet is one without excessive amounts of cold, raw and frozen foods, along with reduced consumption of dairy products and greasy foods. We should also eat foods high in iron, such as spinach, black sweet rice, raisins and dried longan fruit, which enrich Blood. A diet plentiful in freshly cooked vegetables and fish is easily digested and supports the transformation of food into Qi and Blood and ultimately postnatal Essence.

The physical manifestation of Essence is Heavenly Water in women and semen in men. Conception is the union in the womb (called "the baby palace" in TCM) of the red Essence of the mother with the white Essence of the father. Both depend on the healthy functioning of the Kidneys as well as the free, unobstructed movement of Qi and Blood. Since Blood is so fundamental to the female reproductive system, its smooth and sufficient flow is vital to our capacity to conceive. We can tell if our Blood is adequate and moving smoothly if our flow of Heavenly Water is normal. In preparation for conception, then, one of the primary self-care activities we can undertake is to regulate our flow of Heavenly Water. We can do this by following the recommendations given in part two of this book, where we learned that Blood owes its free movement to the proper functioning of the Liver. If the Liver system is balanced, it will facilitate the free flow of Blood and Qi to the Uterus, supporting the Kidney and Spleen networks, and promote the likelihood of pregnancy. Conception can only occur when the Kidneys are strong, the Penetrating Vessel is full of Blood, and the Conception Vessel is open and flowing freely. Eating hot, spicy or greasy foods can impair the free flow of Liver Qi, but the primary cause of Liver Qi Stagnation, as we know, is emotional stress. Even Western medicine acknowledges that stress can have a negative impact on our ability to conceive.

WANDA

Wanda was a small-boned, thin, thirty-five-year-old woman who always had irregular periods. She and her husband wanted to have a baby but weren't able to conceive. Wanda was an interior designer and was often under pressure to meet aggressive deadlines. She had a tendency to bring her work home, literally as well as mentally. One of her projects took her overseas for six months. While she was away, Wanda's flow of Heavenly Water stopped. Her health fell by the wayside as her job consumed her.

When Wanda returned to Canada, she came to see me. "John and I really want to have a baby," she told me. "I've given so much of myself to my job and it hasn't given me what I really want, and in fact it has reduced my chances of having a baby because now my period has stopped. All the effort I put into my work, I want to put into having a family."

The irregularity of her period, coupled with the level of stress she experienced, would make it difficult for her to conceive unless something changed. "This is not another project that you can make happen with your mind," I said to her. "We are holistic beings who are governed by a wisdom that is greater than our minds. Our minds, emotions and bodies are intimately interconnected. The stress you experience at work affects your menstrual flow. Having a child without becoming aware of how you feel and how you deal with your stress would make being a mother another incredibly stressful project, except this time it's for the rest of your life. Learning to handle your emotional life will help restore your period and help this new project begin."

Wanda and I talked about how to develop awareness of when she was stressed, what this felt like in her body and where it was located. Wanda was cut off from her physicality; she resided primarily in her head. We discussed ways that she could relax and deal with her tension. Because she was focused in her mind, on figuring things out, gaining knowledge and solving problems much more so than on feeling or sensing, I suggested she try visualization. This is a guided meditation that uses mental images to clear the mind. Visualizing can be a way to revisit a positive experience or create one. You may wish to try the following simple relaxation visualization exercise:

SIMPLE RELAXATION VISUALIZATION EXERCISE

Settle into a position that feels comfortable. Slowly close your eyes and breathe deeply. Take the time to notice your breathing. Get in touch with your in-breath and your out-breath. Picture a place that is calming and comforting to you—perhaps you've been there with your partner or maybe it's a memory from childhood or maybe it's a place where you've always wanted to go. Often people choose nature to visualize, but wherever you go, go somewhere that is special. Using all your senses, start to experience the details. What does the place look like? Are there lots of colours? Can you hear anything? What are you standing or sitting on? What does it feel like? What is touching your skin? Is the temperature hot or cold? Is there a wind or are you inside? Can you identify any smells? Experience this special place and allow yourself to feel whatever emotions arise. Stay here for as long as you wish; there is no set time to remain. When you wish to leave, breathe deeply a few times. Then gently open your eyes, and slowly take in where you are, notice what is around you.

I also recommended that Wanda do a physical exercise that is effective in helping women to conceive. Sometimes a woman's womb may tilt back, especially if she is in the habit of sleeping on her back. And if she is thin, like Wanda, with little fat tissue to support her Uterus, there is an increased tendency for this to happen, negatively impacting her ability to conceive. The following exercise helps remedy this condition: Kneel and lean your weight forward onto your folded arms on the floor, so that your lower back is at a forty-five-degree angle from the floor (see illustration below). Rest your head on your arms. Hold this position for ten minutes.

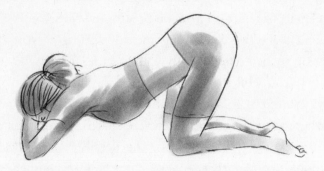

This exercise was also a way for Wanda to connect with her body, specifically her Uterus. She did it once a day faithfully, was careful to rest, eat a proper diet and continue to work on dealing with her stress. Soon her period returned, and about six months later, she became pregnant. She is now the mother of a healthy boy.

Before Wanda could conceive, her Heavenly Water needed to flow again. The regular and normal movement of menstrual Blood is necessary for conception to occur. Since emotional stress has a dramatic impact on the flow of Heavenly Water, it is again the free and appropriate expression of our feelings that is important for the smooth movement of Blood and Qi. Perhaps having a baby, one of our greatest creative projects, brings forth some of our greatest emotional and spiritual resistances. With the possibility of bringing a new being into life, how we see and define ourselves in the world undergoes radical changes. If we are able to move freely with the feelings that arise, there emerges an opening into a new, different and healing way of seeing ourselves. Sometimes, for this to happen, we will need to surrender an old way of being or open to a different choice. Our ability to move with what arises and surrender tightly held beliefs, expectations and identities plays a significant role in our ability to conceive and deliver a healthy newborn.

FALLEN FRUIT

When I became pregnant, my life was unfolding like an ideal script. I was successful in my career as a doctor, my husband and I were considered a perfect match, my family and friends were very supportive of me, and my health was excellent. I was successful in many aspects of my life, and I felt on top of the world.

About six weeks into my pregnancy, I decided to play tennis with some friends. Since this sport is one that I love, that day I played for about four hours. For the next two days, I experienced bleeding and severe cramping in my uterus. I quickly took some Chinese herbs, and then underwent an ultrasound.

To my extreme relief, everything was fine—my baby's heart was beating normally.

Over the next while, I did not engage in any strenuous physical activity—I wanted to get past the first trimester—but I did continue to work at my normal, hectic pace without taking a rest. Around my fourteenth week, I decided to play a light game of tennis with a colleague who was also about three and a half months pregnant; we felt we would be evenly matched. We hadn't seen each other for a few weeks and when we met, my friend thought something was wrong with me—my tummy was as flat as a board. I didn't understand her concern, since I felt well and could feel the fetus moving.

She convinced me to have an ultrasound. As I watched the monitor, I was in shock: there was no heartbeat. The ultrasound revealed that the fetus had shrunk. I couldn't believe it. I vividly remember my colleagues reviewing the ultrasound incredulously, also not comprehending the test results. They called the chairman of the hospital for his opinion. It was very unusual that a fetus would die in the womb without the mother having a fever, heavy bleeding or at least discharge.

Though I felt fine physically, I was going through hell emotionally. Myriad thoughts and emotions bombarded me. My sadness was overwhelming, and I felt a tremendous sense of guilt and self-blame. As a doctor, I should have known what to do to ensure a safe pregnancy and a healthy baby. I felt a deep loss, the loss of my baby and all the hopes and dreams that are born with a child. I felt as if I had lost everything, including my "face." I felt that others would judge me for allowing this to happen and that I had brought much shame to myself. I was left with a huge sense of failure and disappointment.

This feeling of failure was made all the more difficult to endure because, throughout my life, I had excelled at everything I undertook. Whether as a doctor, daughter, sister, wife, friend, student, I had had no experience of not succeeding at what I set out to do. And I had never experienced any serious illness. In hindsight, I realized that I had felt somewhat invincible. Perhaps this was why I hadn't followed the same advice I gave other pregnant women. If one of my patients had cramps and bled like me, I would have advised she take a week off with complete bedrest. Why did I have to pretend everything was OK, even to the point where I felt my colon move and believed it was the fetus moving? I remember my grandmother asking me if a doctor had checked me. I hadn't felt the need to see a doctor, nor did I have time for a medical visit during my busy schedule. And since my family trusted my judgment implicitly, when I said I was doing fine, they were reassured.

I had taken my body for granted in being able to support me. I had driven myself to proceed with my career and other aspects of my life, disregarding any physical constraints that pregnancy brings. I had been confident in my health and my capacity to do it all, and had never thought what my striving for success could mean for my baby. Recognizing how important success was to me helped me to understand that I had unconsciously placed the greatest priority on my career and being a good doctor. After that came my husband, and then a child. This was very difficult for me to acknowledge and made me feel that perhaps I wasn't meant to be a mother. I felt that I was so strongly focused on my career that maybe my baby had sensed it.

I took a month off work and was grateful that my husband, family, friends and colleagues were absolutely supportive of me. I felt no blame from them, only loving care and concern. It was my own judgment and disappointment in myself that brought me the greatest suffering. I came to realize that I had to loosen my grip on my notion of success, be it as a doctor, or as a healthy, competent woman with a strong body. My miscarriage turned out to be a precious gift, in that it introduced me effectively, although painfully, to how I inappropriately defined myself by my success. I really became aware of how my life had been consumed with work and expectations. I remembered how I'd once thought that doctors shouldn't marry. I had believed that their devotion and commitment should be to people who needed healing. I had seen the chairman of my hospital struggle to balance family responsibilities with the demands of his patients. Obviously, I had embodied this belief, and it had revealed itself with my miscarriage.

My loss also equipped me to better understand other women's pain around losing a baby. Women who miscarry need special care and understanding support as they talk about their feelings. An emotional letting go is needed in order for them to heal and move forward with the insights gained.

GLORIA

For Gloria, children were not a priority. Married at age thirty, she had completed a master's degree and was very focused on her career. The traditional concept of settling down had never interested her, and she was not a woman who felt instinctively drawn to babies and children.

It was the death of her father-in-law that ultimately became the catalyst for her and her husband to entertain the idea of pregnancy. After four years of marriage, they decided to try to conceive. Gloria started taking hormones to enhance her fertility. After five months she became pregnant. At the sixth week, she miscarried. Three months later, she became pregnant again. She saw an obstetrician and two days later started spotting. Within the week, she miscarried.

Gloria felt frantic and was extremely bloated from water retention. It was at this point that she came to my clinic. Because of the large amount of hormones she'd been taking, she needed to detoxify and cleanse. I put her on a two-week vegetable fast, and then started to strengthen her body through acupuncture treatment and herbs. As well, she had to emotionally transition from being a career-focused woman to being a mother. In less than six months, Gloria became pregnant once more. This time, happily, she was able to carry the fetus to full term, and deliver a beautiful, healthy girl.

Two years later, when Gloria was thirty-eight, she and her husband decided to have another child. She became pregnant in June but miscarried in August. Six months later, she was again pregnant, but around the twelfth week, began spotting and miscarried. Within six months, Gloria conceived once more. However, at six weeks she had an ultrasound, and no heartbeat was detected. Gloria was extremely depressed; she had had three miscarriages over a sixteen-month period. Adding to her depression was the pressure she felt to have a second child before her fortieth birthday. After forty, she was afraid she would be too old to parent. The milestone was a heavy burden for her.

I suggested to Gloria that she let go of the need to have a baby by the age of forty. Gloria says that when she relinquished that deadline for herself, she became pregnant again and eventually gave birth to a healthy baby boy.

Upon conception, the flow of Heavenly Water ceases and Blood transforms into Essence to nurture the fetus and the mother. Postnatal Essence is extracted from food and fluids by the Spleen and Stomach. Overconsumption of cold, raw or sweet foods, along with emotional imbalances such as excessive worry or overthinking, can impair the Spleen's and Stomach's ability to generate and then transport Blood. If this happens, the flow of Blood to the Uterus may be obstructed or slowed down.

Our capacity to hold on to preconceived thoughts and feelings can block our flow of Qi and Blood. Energetically, we constrict and tighten. How often has each of us, unable to vent our feelings, felt a hard knot forming in our belly? This knot is a physical manifestation of Stagnant emotions, Qi. Emotional, mental or spiritual inner conflict can cause energy to stagnate in the Meridians and Organs. Depending on the duration or intensity of this energetic blockage, the Stagnation may be expressed in a physical symptom or condition, or may undermine our vitality in some other aspects of life. I had needed to let go of my fear of failure and my drive for success. Gloria had had to release herself from her self-identity as a career professional and then her need to be pregnant before she reached forty. In each instance, letting go was a significant aspect of healing into a future pregnancy.

SECOND CHANCE

Three years after my miscarriage, I conceived again. I was excited but also anxious. Would I be able to have a good pregnancy? Would I deliver a healthy baby? Of course, I felt considerable pressure because of my previous miscarriage. This time I was careful not to engage in heavy exercise for the first trimester. During the first three months, the energy of the Kidneys and Liver is especially important. They must be healthy and vital. If the energy of these Organs is not optimal, the fetus is extremely vulnerable to injury. When I reached the twelfth week, I felt confident that I had passed the critical time for a miscarriage. My body felt strong and had settled into being pregnant.

My husband and I lived in a six-storey apartment building that did not have an elevator—like the vast majority of apartment buildings in China. I returned home from work one day on my bicycle and decided that I would carry it up the five flights of stairs to our apartment. Five minutes after I arrived home, I felt something hot winding down my legs like a snake. I looked down and screamed. Blood was coursing out of my body and into my socks. I was paralyzed with fear and my husband had to carry me to bed. Within a short time, the bed was soaked with blood. I was taken to the emergency room, given medication and sent home with strict instructions for bedrest.

This time, I remained in bed for two to three weeks. I was so afraid I'd lose this baby I kept saying to my fetus over and over again, "Please stay, I won't do that again." I had challenged my body a second time, believing it was stronger than it was. I lived a healthy life, didn't smoke or drink, ate a nutritious and balanced diet and worked at what I loved. In my mind, this somehow gave me the excuse to work my body harder. On one level, I had harmony in my life, but on another level, I was out of balance, pushing my limits. My mind was in the driver's seat, and was forcing my body to do more than it could handle. I expected so much from my body, wanting it to be tough and strong, wanting it to do what my mind asked of it. I came to realize that I had to make a deal with myself: I would take care of my body, and it wouldn't give me any trouble.

Learning that my mind didn't have ultimate control was a huge lesson. My experiences with my pregnancies enabled me to surrender and let go of the need for control. I began a new relationship with myself, which was healthier as well as more balanced on all levels.

There is a Buddhist fable that shows how we can hold on to our beliefs and not even be aware that we are doing so. One day, a young monk said to an older monk, "Our vows of celibacy are very grave vows." The older monk agreed. The young monk added, "And we also vow not to be in the company of women." The older monk agreed once again, and then pointed to a woman standing on the bank of the river who was dressed in wedding clothes.

"And what of that woman who will miss her sister's wedding ceremony if someone doesn't carry her across the water?"

"Oh, rules are rules and not to be broken," said the novice monk, who had recently learned all the rules.

"And what of compassion?" asked the senior monk. "Look at her. She is very upset, and if we don't help her, she will not be able to attend her sister's wedding."

"We have our rules."

Without saying another word, the older monk gathered the woman in his arms, waded through the water and set her on the distant shore. When he returned, the two monks continued their journey in silence.

After half a day had passed, the young monk said, "I don't think it was right that you picked up that beautiful young woman and carried her across the river."

The older monk replied, "Dear monk, I set that young woman down on the bank half a day ago. It seems you've been carrying her since that time."

Pregnancy is an opportunity to reconnect with our bodies, hearts, minds and spirits. We are asked to surrender to the changes that occur. We must trust in this natural process that prepares us for an even greater letting go—childbirth.

CHAPTER TWELVE

Ripening the Fruit

Having a baby brings with it tremendous changes, physically, emotionally and spiritually, within a very short period of time. For 100 per cent of the pregnant women I have treated, their emotional state and their attitudes towards having a baby and what this means to them as women had a deep impact on the nature of their pregnancies. Women who resisted gaining weight, fearing loss of control over their bodies, or identified too strongly with their physical appearance struggled against the natural flow and growth of creating a child.

Essence and the Blood and Qi of the mother nourishes and assists in the development of the fetus in the womb. Therefore, how a mother takes care of herself during her pregnancy has a profound effect on the development and health of her baby.

OLIVIA

Olivia was in shock when I suggested she was pregnant. She said, "It can't be, I just had my period last week." Olivia did not want to be pregnant again. She had had a very difficult eight years with her two daughters, who had experienced very poor health, and she had finally reached a point in her life where she felt rested, healthy and fit.

When Olivia was pregnant with Gabriela, her first child, it was a difficult time. She and her husband, Victor, were living in Mexico, having fled the civil war in El Salvador, and their diet consisted mainly of beans and corn. In trying to ensure that her younger brother got safely out of Mexico, Olivia had had to refuse an invitation to come to Canada as a refugee. She was fortunate that Canada extended a rare second invitation and that she and her family were able to move to Toronto.

Four years after their immigration, Olivia became pregnant with her second child, Isabel. At the time, Victor was struggling with high cholesterol, and Gabriela was suffering from severe asthma attacks. Olivia felt anxious and was suspicious of the "system" in Canada. She said, "I am never sure if my personal information is being monitored or how it might be used against me. Perhaps these are old fears coming from the oppressive regime I lived under in Central America."

During this pregnancy, Olivia ate whatever she could; she always felt hungry and craved food to fill her up. She lived by the adage that she was "eating for two," not realizing that this meant she should eat the quality necessary for two, not the quantity. Olivia would wake up in the middle of the night and eat whatever she could find in the refrigerator. When it was time to deliver her baby, Olivia had a very difficult labour, and Isabel arrived black and blue in colour.

Over the next four years, as each of the girls was sick with asthma, allergies and childhood illnesses, Olivia grew very tired.

Adapting to a new country, going to school and taking care of her sick daughters day and night had exhausted her to the point where her health was suffering. One afternoon, as she was driving home after taking Isabel to the hospital the previous night, she saw a car rushing towards her but had no energy to react. She said, "I just watched and let the car hit me."

Soon after the accident, I started to treat the entire family. Over time, Olivia lost the weight she had gained during her pregnancies and was less tired. She was delighted that her daughters were no longer having asthma attacks or suffering from allergies. As well, Victor's cholesterol levels had decreased. For Olivia, the change in her family's and her own well-being was such a welcome relief that she didn't want to be pregnant again.

I asked her if she wanted a boy. She said yes. Jokingly, I told her that if she had a boy, she could keep him, and that if she had a girl, I would keep her and look after her. She told me that if she was going to have this baby, she definitely did not want another sick child. Olivia made a conscious decision to have a healthy pregnancy and a healthy baby, and to follow my recommendations.

I first suggested that Olivia try to watch her weight, since gaining too much would not be healthy for either her or her baby. Excess weight can contribute to high blood pressure, cholesterol and a difficult labour. I asked Olivia to reduce the amount of coffee she drank and helped her to establish a diet with lots of fresh fruit and vegetables, fish and nuts. Victor often said that he thought Olivia would give birth to a guinea pig or rabbit because of all the carrots and lettuce she ate.

Olivia felt she could trust me since we were both recent

immigrants and had previously survived under similar repressive governments. She said that it was very important for her to have me to talk to and didn't feel anxious as a result. For Olivia, this was an important healing step. Allowing me to assist and guide her reassured her that everything would be OK, or at least could be handled or managed.

Olivia went full term with an easy pregnancy and delivered a beautiful, healthy baby girl. Alyssa is a very different child than her two older sisters. Though Olivia waited for her third daughter to develop asthma or become ill like her first two, Alyssa never did. In addition, she has a very different physical and energetic structure than Gabriela and Isabel. She is thin, lean and full of energy, while her two sisters are heavier, and physically and energetically less active.

How we and our partners take care of ourselves is a significant consideration in the constitution of our children. Olivia and Victor were very healthy and not fatigued when they conceived Alyssa. As well, during her pregnancy, Olivia took care to maintain a proper and supportive diet. She also dealt with deep emotional issues by letting go of her distrust and opening up to another person. When pregnant, it is important that we pay attention to our level of stress. We should watch where we hold on and resist the flow of energy in our emotions and in our body. We should try not to overwork and get fatigued. As we build our energy, we will have that much more to pass on to our children. The state of our emotional, mental and spiritual health, along with our dietary habits and lifestyle choices, have far-reaching implications and tremendous impact on the ease of our pregnancies, as well as the future health of our children. We may not have a great deal of say in the evolution of our physiology during pregnancy and child-birth, but we can exert significant influence on the overall vitality and character of our children.

NURTURING ZHAO ZHAO

In China, pregnancy is regarded as a normal and expected phase of a married woman's life and there are certain practices that are followed. According to Chinese tradition, what a preg-nant woman does, sees, experiences and feels will affect her unborn child. Thoughts are associated with the Heart Organ system, and what affects a woman's mind will impact her Heart and influence her unborn baby through Blood. Upon conception, then, a woman talks to her baby, reads good books, listens to music and massages her tummy. She doesn't lose her temper or get too sad. During the early stages of preg-nancy, she relaxes, rests, refrains from heavy lifting and main-tains a proper diet to guarantee a healthy pregnancy and a healthy baby.

When I was pregnant with Zhao Zhao, I didn't experience morning sickness, but I have treated many women who were nauseous and vomited during their pregnancy. Some women are sick only when they wake up in the morning; for others, the smell of a certain food can make them feel nauseous; for still others, nausea is worse later in the day, and many women experience queasiness throughout the entire day. Many women find that morning sickness passes after the first trimester, while others suffer with it for their entire pregnancy. Nausea is a result of Stomach Qi that is blocked and unable to flow in its regular downward direction and moves upwards instead. There are various causes of this counterflow of Stomach Qi, including eating cold, raw and frozen foods and drinking cold fluids, overworrying, overworking, being exhausted or experiencing emotional stress. All these factors can produce imbalances in the Meridians that impact the flow of Stomach Qi. It is of the utmost importance that we try to normalize and equalize this flow as much as possible during pregnancy by changing our dietary habits, getting rest, avoiding overtaxing ourselves mentally and trying not to be obsessive in our thinking.

We should also drink lots of fluids and reduce the amount of processed foods that we consume. Ginger is an herb that is very helpful in treating nausea. We can make tea with fresh ginger, mint and honey or, if preferred, with fresh ginger and orange peel.

Ginger and Mint Tea
Makes 8 servings

1-inch piece	fresh ginger root, peeled and grated
5 leaves	fresh mint
4 cups	boiling water
Honey to taste	

1. Place ginger and mint in a teapot.
2. Pour boiling water over ginger and mint. Cover and allow to steep for 3 to 5 minutes before serving. Add honey to taste.

Ginger and Orange Tea
Makes 8 servings

1-inch piece	fresh ginger root, peeled and grated
1/2 tablespoon	grated orange rind
4 cups	boiling water

Honey to taste

1. Place ginger and grated orange peel in a teapot.
2. Pour boiling water over ginger and orange peel. Cover and allow to steep for 3 to 5 minutes before serving. Add honey to taste.

Alternatively, fresh ginger can be sliced into one-and-a-half-inch circles and taped to the insides of the wrists and over-top the navel. These are the same anti-nausea acupuncture points that "sea bands," which are wristbands worn to counter seasickness, target. Another way to use ginger to treat morning sickness is to eat ginger rice.

Ginger Rice
Makes 1 serving

1	large, fresh ginger root
1 cup	rice

1. Peel ginger root, and cut it up into rough chunks. Place the ginger in a bowl, and with a hand blender, mash it up. Put the mashed ginger in a piece of cheesecloth and squeeze out the ginger juice into

the bowl. You should have 1 teaspoon of ginger
juice.

2. Put the rice in a medium skillet over low heat.
Sprinkle the ginger juice over the rice, and stir-fry
it until the rice turns yellow, about 5 minutes.
Chewing the rice will help alleviate nausea.

When I was pregnant with Zhao Zhao, I was careful to eat
foods that supported his growth and development in utero. I
ate many kinds of nuts and seeds, especially walnuts,
almonds and sesame seeds. These are considered "brain
food," since they contain essential fats that the brain needs in
order to properly develop. Interestingly, one half of a walnut
looks like a brain or kidney, and walnuts are thought to
increase Kidney Qi. Walnuts are also beneficial for the development of the spinal cord. Fish, also because of its beneficial
oil, is another food that I ate more of during my pregnancy.

I regularly drank soup made from lots of beef, pork or
chicken bones. I consumed many, many gallons of this soup
to help prevent cramps and also for the formation of Zhao
Zhao's teeth and bones. To best extract the calcium out of
the bones, add two tablespoons of apple cider vinegar to the
soup. In China, milk, including soy milk, is not used as a
source of calcium, since it is believed to lead to the formation of Dampness that can impede the smooth flow of Qi.

Bone Soup
Makes 6 servings

2 pounds	beef, pork or chicken bones
10 cups	cold water
2 tablespoons	apple cider vinegar

1. Place bones in a large pot. Add 10 cups cold water and apple cider vinegar. Bring to boil. Cover and reduce heat; simmer for 4 hours.

As our volume of Blood increases during the term of a pregnancy, it is important to eat foods that nourish and support Blood. Some good choices are eggs, raisins, walnuts, dried longan fruit, black sweet rice, spinach and other leafy green vegetables. In Kunming, the city where I lived, there is, fortunately, an abundance of fresh vegetables and fruits year-round. I ate much fresh produce during my pregnancy and took special care to eat high-fibre vegetables, like mustard greens, to counter constipation. I also ate a mixture of pine nuts and honey. This can be made by soaking pine nuts in raw honey for two weeks, then eating one teaspoon every day (see recipe on next page). Other self-care practices helpful in preventing or reducing constipation are drinking lots of water—about eight glasses a day—eating moderate amounts of food regularly, reducing salt intake and engaging in regular exercise, such as walking.

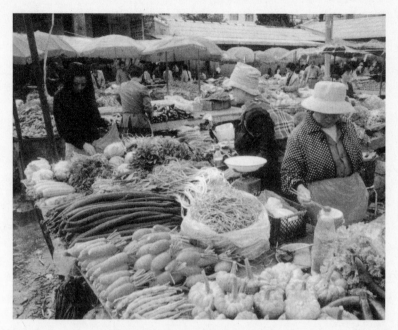

An outdoor vegetable market in Kunming

Honeyed Pine Nuts

1 cup   pine nuts
Raw honey

1. Put pine nuts in a jar with a lid and add enough raw
   honey to cover. Screw on lid and store the jar in the
   cupboard for 2 weeks.

Walking also helps with edema, or water retention. Later
in my pregnancy I prevented edema from worsening by sitting
with my legs raised above my waist at the end of the day.
Edema, coupled with high blood pressure, can be very serious,

so a medical doctor should be consulted for treatment and follow-up. You should also visit a doctor if you experience dizziness or diarrhea. Self-care for edema includes reducing salt intake, reducing consumption of dairy and greasy foods, drinking lots of water and eating small amounts frequently—about five to six times a day. In addition, it is helpful to massage the Spleen acupuncture point, San Yin Jiao, located on the inside of the lower leg, approximately four finger widths above the ankle (see page 97). Massage this point twenty times.

Sexual intercourse is to be avoided during the first trimester. The Kidney and Liver Qi are not strong and firm yet, and the fetus is susceptible to physical trauma and upset, as well as emotional injury. It is also recommended that we not have sex after the seventh month.

To prevent back pain, I did regular stretching. One helpful exercise is to kneel on our hands and knees on the floor, in a position resembling a table (see illustration below). Our arms should be straight and underneath our shoulders, and our knees should be directly underneath our hips. Inhale slowly, and as we exhale, we tighten our tummy and arch our back

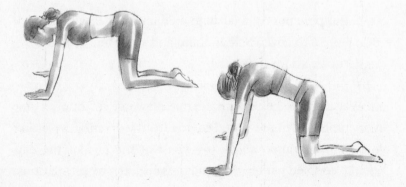

upwards. We relax our back and tummy as we inhale and return to our original position. Repeat several times slowly.

To alleviate lower back pain, we can also rub our hands together until we feel heat, and place each of them over our Kidneys, which are located just above the waist on either side of the spine (see illustration at left). Often, the strain on our backs makes it difficult to sleep at night. I found that sleeping on my side with a pillow placed between my knees was one way of being a little more comfortable during the later stages of my pregnancy. Sleeping on the right side is considered best, as it allows the Stomach to freely drain into the Intestines. Additionally, it does not put undue or excessive pressure on the Heart.

Insomnia may be a problem during pregnancy and can be helped by trying to maintain a regular sleep schedule. We can try to relax before retiring, and slow our mind down before going to sleep. Meditation, listening to music, quietly reading or a warm shallow bath may help us unwind from a busy day. Massaging our temples may also help relax us. We may try massaging the acupuncture point Yong Quan, or Bubbling Spring, which is located on the sole of each foot at the depression below the ball of the foot (see page 96). Apply a firm downward motion with the thumb or knuckles to the hollow, with pressure directed inwards and towards the big toes. Apply pressure for one minute. We can also place this part of the foot firmly on a small book or stone to stimulate this acupuncture point.

In order to prepare myself for breastfeeding my baby, three months before my delivery date, I began to regularly grasp my nipples and pull them out. Initially, breastfeeding may not be as natural a process as we think when we see a mother nursing her baby. A newborn has a sucking instinct but will need help latching on to the mother's nipples. Pulling them out helps extend the nipples and give the baby something to really suck on. Also, I took a damp new towel or firm sponge and brushed each nipple for almost five minutes daily. This helped get my nipples ready so that they wouldn't be tender and sore when I started breastfeeding.

In my seventh month, I developed brown spots on my face. These are generally a result of Liver Qi and Blood Stagnation, and in the West, are often referred to as liver spots. Herbs, such as *Xiao Yao Wan* and *Dong Quai,* which are often recommended to release stuck Liver Qi, can be effective in reducing the formation of these spots. These patent remedies are available at Chinese herbal pharmacies, however I would only advise taking these at the suggestion of a TCM practitioner. We should also try to avoid the sun, since it stimulates the formation and progression of liver spots.

If symptoms arise during pregnancy, address these as quickly as possible. Correcting imbalances will ensure that Organ function is not impaired and the baby's health, as well as our own, will be better supported. Acupuncture is generally applied to deal with certain conditions, such as edema and morning sickness, or to support the healthy functioning of any weakened Organ systems that are not sustaining the fetus. However, care must be taken not to massage or needle acupuncture points that will stimulate the fetus or the Organs in the abdominal area. During gestation, the fetus should be resting and not be excited. In Chinese medicine, pregnancy is said to last ten months based on the lunar calendar (approximately nine months in the solar calendar). During each of the ten months of gestation, one specific Organ network nourishes the fetus.

In addition, there are specific self-care measures we can take each month to support ourselves and our babies throughout the pregnancy. An understanding of our baby's month-by-month development helps to harmonize our daily activities with our baby's needs.

PREGNANCY CALENDAR

The information in Table 5 on the following pages comes from ancient texts and relates to the development of the fetus during each of the ten months of gestation in the lunar calendar. Pregnancy is also shown from a Western medicine perspective.

TABLE 5: PREGNANCY CALENDAR

CHINESE MEDICINE*

Month (Lunar)	Related Channel	Description
1	Liver	• The embryo is sustained through the mother's Liver Channel.
2	Gallbladder	• The embryo is sustained through the mother's Gallbladder Channel • Original Qi (Prenatal Essence / *Yuan Qi*) manifests. • As the embryo grows, the mother may feel joint pain.
3	Pericardium	• The fetus is sustained through the mother's Heart Channel. • The sex and shape of the body of the fetus is still to be determined based on the factors influencing the mother.

*Giovanni Maciocia, *Obstetrics and Gynecology in Chinese Medicine* (Edinburgh: Churchill Livingstone, 1998), 9.

Self-Care	Month (Solar)	WESTERN MEDICINE Description
• Circulation of Blood is weakened, so avoid physical over-exertion. • Eat cooked foods that are easy to digest. • Sour foods are allowed if a craving develops. • Avoid extreme heat (which may make the fetus fearful) and cold (which translates as pain for the fetus).	1	• After implantation, the umbilical cord and placenta form. • Sex is determined. • The heart, lungs, brain and nervous system start to form. • The brain, eyes, mouth, inner ear and digestive tract start to form. • Around the 25th day, the heart begins to beat. • Spots for eyes, ears and nose are present. • "Buds" for limbs are forming.
• Avoid hot, pungent foods. • Refrain from sexual intercourse. • Avoid overwork. • Avoid extreme cold (which may provoke miscarriage) and heat (which may weaken the fetus).	2	• Major organs are beginning to form. • The embryo's elbows, knees, toes, fingers and sexual organs develop. • Bones start to harden. • The spinal cord appears. • Eyelids are formed but closed. • The inner ear begins to develop.
• To have a son, the mother should practise shooting arrows. • If a daughter is desired, the mother should hold jewellery. • To have a beautiful child, the mother should look at jade. • For a child with a good heart, the mother should sit quietly as much as possible.	3	• Soft nails develop on fingers and toes. • Hair begins to grow. • Kidneys form and deliver urine to the bladder. • The baby's sex becomes apparent. • The fetus's organs are completely formed by the end of the third month.

CHINESE MEDICINE		
Month (Lunar)	**Related Channel**	**Description**
4	Triple Burner	• The fetus is sustained through the mother's Small Intestine Channel. • The fetus starts to absorb Essence from the Kidneys of the mother to develop blood vessels. • The Yang organs are formed.
5	Spleen	• The fetus is sustained through the mother's Spleen Channel. • The temperament of the fetus develops from the mother's essential Qi of the Heart. • Arms and legs form.
6	Stomach	• The fetus is sustained through the mother's Stomach Channel. • Sinew develops from the mother's Lung Qi. • Mouth and eyes form.
7	Lungs	• The fetus is sustained through the mother's Lung Channel. • Bones form from the mother's essential Liver Qi. • Hair and skin form.

| Self-Care | WESTERN MEDICINE | |
	Month (Solar)	Description
• Eating fish, rice or wild geese will strengthen the fetus's Qi and Blood, ensure the eyes and ears are bright and sensitive, and keep the Small Intestine Channel free and clear. • Moderate the amount of food eaten. • Mother should be calm and avoid emotional distress.	4	• The fetus's skin is transparent and thin. • Hair, eyebrows and eyelashes form. • Twenty buds for baby teeth form. • Vocal cords form. • The fetus is able to suck its thumb. • All limbs are completely formed. • The skin is covered in fine hair, referred to as lanugo.
• Sleep for long periods. • Keep warm. • Go out in the sun. • Eat beef, wheat and lamb. • Take care not to eat too little or too much.	5	• Hair, eyebrows and eyelashes begin to grow. • The fetus is asleep and awake at regular intervals. • The fetus grows muscle.
• Engage in light exercise. • Go outdoors. • To ensure strong sinew and muscle, firm spine and back, eat meat from wild animals and look at dogs and horses running. • Eat moderate amounts of sweet foods.	6	• A white substance called vernix covers the skin. • The brain is quickly developing. • Females develop eggs in their ovaries. • Lungs are not fully developed yet.
• Exercise (extend and flex joints) to stimulate Blood and Qi circulation. • Eat rice to support the fetus's bones and teeth. • Do not eat cold foods. • Keep warm.	7	• Bones start to harden and grow strong. • A layer of fat forms under the skin. • Lanugo disappears from the face. • The brain and nervous system grow rapidly. • The testicles start to move down into the scrotum.

CHINESE MEDICINE		
Month (Lunar)	**Related Channel**	**Description**
8	Large Intestine	• The fetus is sustained through the mother's Large Intestine Channel. • Skin growth is encouraged by receiving the mother's essential Spleen Qi.
9	Kidneys	• The fetus is sustained through the mother's Kidney Channel. • Skin and hair growth is nourished by the mother's Essence received. • All Organs are formed.
10	Bladder	• The fetus is sustained through the mother's Bladder Channel. • The Yin Organs are fully developed. • The Yang Organs are without obstructions.

| Self-Care | WESTERN MEDICINE | |
	Month (Solar)	Description
• Avoid emotional disturbances. • The mother's Qi is maintained through quiet breathing practice, which promotes luxuriant skin in the fetus. • Do not overeat. • Avoid getting angry.	8	• The brain continues to quickly develop. • The baby is mature enough now to survive if born. • Eyes are open. • The baby may move into position for birth.
• Eat sweet foods. • Stay away from damp environments. • Wear clothing that is loose. • Speak softly.	9	• The baby is fully developed. • The bones in the head are flexible and soft for delivery. • Most of the lanugo has disappeared.
• To encourage the baby's mental abilities and the development of joints, the mother should focus her Qi three finger widths below her naval at the Lower *Dan Tian*.		

CHAPTER THIRTEEN

The Labour of Letting Go

The day before I was born, my mother stayed at her office after work until midnight to study the teachings of the Communist government. She did this every night because the government exerted pressure on its citizens to do so, and even encouraged people to watch each other and report any counter-revolutionary activities they suspected. When my mother arrived home, her contractions started. My father was away on a business trip at the time, and my sisters and brother were asleep. My mother did not want to wake them, so she quietly slipped out and went upstairs to ask her neighbour to walk her to the hospital.

During labour, my mother did not cry out, or yell, or in fact make any noise. She said that despite the pain, she felt an inner strength and didn't feel the need to scream or cry. She also said that my father wasn't there to hear her anyway and thought that if she made too much noise, the nurses would tire of her. The other women in the ward thought my mother had a pain-free delivery, and speculated that she had studied Russian women, who, reputedly, had babies without any pain.

How my mother dealt with my birth was a reflection of how she lived her life and continues to live her life today. Childbirth is a milestone in the feminine life cycle that she was able to move through as it naturally unfolded. She did not spend a lot of time worrying about what was going to happen. She had not been conditioned to view childbirth with foreboding and fear. My mother was confident in her ability and strength to work through the pain and process of giving birth.

Women throughout time have given birth to healthy infants who have grown to have children of their own. And yet childbirth is still viewed with anxiety, fear and apprehension. Is this a result of our concern around the health of our babies, or fear around pain? Is it nervousness that we'll do something wrong or that something will go wrong? Is it our fear over the loss of our ability to control what is happening with our minds? Or is it the result of a general lack of confidence in natural processes and a distrust of our innate wisdom? I often wonder to what degree medicated technological deliveries have separated us from what should be a natural birthing experience. Could focusing on what could go wrong contribute to our distrust of our bodies' intelligence of this event? I do not deny the value and benefits of modern medicine, but I think it's important that we reconnect with the inner wisdom of the female body. This is the same intelligence that our body accesses when it "knows" how to heal a cut. Trusting in this wisdom will help reduce our anxiety around the uncertainties of childbirth and may ease our labour. Though we can neither predict what will happen nor control it, we can learn to be with our uncertainty in a new way. In order for something new to be born into our lives, we must experience something unfamiliar.

One way to deal with the unknown is to be prepared and understand how we can trust our own internal resources and coping skills. Becoming aware of the confidence we have in ourselves to deal with unpredictable and stressful situations may give us a clue as to how we may respond during labour. How have I reacted in the past when I've been in a situation that is unfamiliar and physically painful? How much belief did I have in my ability to handle the situation or person? What inner resources did I call upon to help me?

In reflecting on these questions, I realize that the trust I have in my inner resources often struggles for air time with all the other voices that say: "You're doing the wrong thing"; "There'll be a reprisal for your behaviour"; "What an embarrassment you are"; "You're not strong enough or smart enough or caring enough or professional enough." How quick I am to discount who I am, subjugate what it is I want or trivialize what I believe in. I am given to judging my motivations and behaviour and am harsh on myself. All of this erodes trust in myself.

Believing in myself is to trust my inner resources, an inherent intelligence that resides within each of us. How do I honour my feelings, and how do I value my intuition? Connecting with this inner intelligence is connecting with Yin energy, the feminine. It is to trust that inkling I have about a person, to listen to that hunch I have around a situation or to pay attention to the ache in my heart. To nourish self-confidence, which is none other than our inner intelligence, I must make space for what it is that I really want to emerge. I must develop a relationship with my body and feelings, and learn to nurture what is best for me. In doing so, I honour and respect the deeply intuitive voice that is our collective wisdom, the wisdom that knows how to give birth. In trusting our bodies' knowing of the birth process, we lessen the anxiety and fear around the uncertainties of childbirth. This natural event has a miraculous design that is already being enacted, if only we can give ourselves over to it.

Besides empowering ourselves with confidence in our bodies' innate wisdom to work with the unknown, we can seek knowledge about the various stages of the birthing process by attending prenatal classes. Knowledge of how a contraction develops and peaks, plus an overview of our physiology and anatomy, will prepare us to work with our bodies as best as we can and participate in the delivery, rather than feel powerless. If we have no idea what is happening to our bodies during childbirth, we may feel anxious and afraid, and this often increases the intensity of any pain we are experiencing and creates stress for our babies.

We can nurture our self-confidence around childbirth by working with the intimate relationship between mind and body. Using visualization techniques to affect our mental, emotional and physical states helps us through the uncertainties of labour, and helps us to relax so that we may tap into our inner wisdom. Since the mind and body are connected, practices such as visualization and meditation can have a positive impact on our physical condition, our experience and reactions.

VISUALIZATION

Creative visualization may involve imagining in detail the way you'd like to give birth and what your labour and delivery will be like. Develop a clear picture of a safe labour and a healthy baby, and whatever else you may wish. Identifying what you truly want and believe is possible is an important first step in creating your visualization. Select images that you are comfortable and familiar with. When you have an idea of what it is you want and have the pictures clear in your mind, always imagine them as if they have already happened, rather than as a wish or desire. Your visualization may involve picturing where you will deliver your baby: At home? In the hospital? In water? What does the room look like? What music will be playing? Who will be there? How long will your labour be? How will you ride each contraction?

You may decide to work with metaphoric images in your visualization. Pick symbolic images that are meaningful to you so that your mind understands the connection. If you want your cervix to open easily and gently, you may choose to visualize a flower unfolding from a bud, opening its petals into full bloom. Metaphoric images can often be the most powerful in a visualization and may serve to ease the process and thereby lessen the stress of anticipated events.

You may wish to start your visualization practice early in your pregnancy, so that when you go into labour it will appear with the ease and calm born of familiarity. Try to bring your visualization to mind every day. You may find that taking a few deep in- and out-breaths is helpful in relaxing your body before you begin to visualize.

Developing visualizations of the childbirth experience does not mean that we ignore the possibility that the unexpected or pain may arise. What this practice does is help develop positive images of childbirth to replace previously frightening or negative images. We may visualize giving birth as a natural event that is not fraught with danger or the need for medical intervention. By creating our own picture of childbirth, we are more apt to trust the wisdom of our bodies and develop the self-confidence to deliver our babies in accordance with nature, thereby making the entire process a more positive one.

MEDITATION

Meditation is very helpful in relaxing our bodies and calming our minds. It can nurture trust in our inner knowing and reduce many of the fears related to childbirth. Connecting with the natural order of the world, taking time to recognize the cycles and cadence of nature may also help us to value and honour our own natures.

We may meditate on the sound of the water's song as it dances over rocks, or the feeling of the wind caressing our bodies with coolness as the sun heats our skin with its penetrating rays, or the smell of the fresh, invigorating air after a spring downpour. In these moments there is nothing to do, no place to go, nothing to understand and no decisions to make. Try to slow down and feel the harmony and peace of nature. Allow this to permeate your body and release you from your thoughts, beliefs and attitudes for this moment. Surrender to

rgy moving through your body and absorb the deep
ion it offers. Each of these meditations can wind their
nto your body and relieve the tensions that have been
flooding your mind and interfering with the relative ease of
this natural yet unfamiliar process.

We can also deal with negative energies through a varia-
tion on the Buddhist practice of Tonglen. In Tibetan, *Tonglen*
means "giving and receiving." It is practised to help summon
compassion for ourselves in our fear and suffering. Tonglen
opens our hearts to what is blocking us from connecting
deeply with our true nature. In helping us to break through
the obstructions that keep us from trusting our inner wisdom, we discover a new relationship with what gives us pain
and stress.

In order to open our hearts, Tonglen teaches us to move
close to that which brings us suffering. We do not try to get rid
of our pain, but rather move in to touch the centre of it. By
keeping our minds and hearts open as we breathe with our
feelings of fear, or whatever else may be present, we begin to
see how our hearts and minds are closed related to fear.
Tonglen is a practice to get to know the feelings as felt qualities in our bodies, and then allow them to transform without
embarking on an endless journey of suffering. We may feel
fear about what may happen during our labour, and before we
realize it, we are off imagining the worst possible scenarios.
Setting off on this tangent causes us great distress. Tonglen
helps us to let go of this chain reaction.

It is said that the seeds of compassion are sown in the
fields of our neuroses, fears and what we consider to be negative, as is trust, relaxation and the development of inner

strength to ease us through childbirth. There is value in our pain, if we allow transformative energies to arise and effectively work with it. This view is embodied in the concept of Yin and Yang, which holds that the roots of compassion will be found in our difficult emotions, and the source of what are generally considered negative feelings are in compassion.

There is no need to eradicate our fear. We can use it as an object of mindfulness, not judging it as good or bad, right or wrong, but simply touching it, then letting it go. The experience of fear in itself is not unhealthy. It is rather our continued or excessive reaction to the arising of this normal human emotion that is the cause of disease. If we can develop a healthy way to be with our fear so that we are not left in an empty state without an emotional experience, we will facilitate the free flow of Qi. Tonglen is a useful practice to become intimate with the raw energy of our difficult feelings so that we may transform our relationship with these emotions.

A TONGLEN MEDITATION

- Sit in meditation and focus on your true nature; you may think of this as collective wisdom or enlightened compassion or your Higher Self.
- Now reflect on a feeling that is uncomfortable or difficult; perhaps it is the fear that sometimes accompanies thoughts of childbirth. Move into the middle of your discomfort and pain. You may feel an automatic response to push the fear away or resist and do something so you won't have to feel. Notice this and breathe in your discomfort, knowing that what you are feeling is felt by millions of other women.

- As you pay attention to this feeling, start to become aware of the suffering that this emotion has brought you. Make a mental note of the stress and worry that you've experienced because of your fear. Perhaps your sleeping has become disturbed, or your temper short. Now, begin to sense a tenderness and caring for this part of yourself that fears.
- Begin to breathe in this difficult feeling as black, heavy smoke or a dark cloud. Breathe it in through all the pores in your body.
- Then breathe out white, cool, refreshing light that has the nature of inspiration, spaciousness, loving joy and letting go. Send this to the part of yourself that is in pain and suffers from the fear. Exhale through every pore in your body.
- If your thoughts distract you, note them without getting involved and transform them into dark smoke.
- Notice if your breath is longer and deeper with the inhalation or the exhalation. Is it easier for you to give or to receive?
- Continue to give and receive as you breathe for as long as you feel comfortable. As your practice deepens and you become increasingly familiar with your feelings, so too will your level of comfort and confidence.

In practising Tonglen, we make friends with our difficult emotions and are then able to stay with all that arises. By moving close to our fears, we open our hearts to ourselves, and compassion arises not only for us but for others as well. We may be relieved of the fear of childbirth or at least become more familiar with it, so that it does not have such power to constrict us. It helps us to relax and prepares us to work with the challenges and powerful energy of childbirth.

SUPPORT PEOPLE

Sharing the childbirth experience with support people—partners, family, friends—is another way we can help ourselves work with our fears and anxieties around childbirth. Involving support people in the process is reassuring on a number of levels and will help many women who are afraid of being alone during childbirth.

Allowing ourselves to depend upon our family members and friends will help us to build trust, as well as to accept support. We extend the birthing experience to more than one individual; we do not have to be strong and do this alone, or feel abandoned, isolated and on our own. Receiving others' assistance during this time of great unknowns invites us to be vulnerable to them and, ultimately, to trust them. In so doing, we surrender to a process that is our great creative power, our collective wisdom, as well as our collective and united strength.

ACUPRESSURE

One way to include support people in your labour is to get them to massage your acupressure points. To deliver a baby, Qi must descend. Pregnancy involves accumulating Yin—Blood—while labour and delivery represents a shift to active Yang energy, which is needed to discharge the baby and Blood. Acupressure will assist Qi in moving downwards, and is a safe, noninvasive and effective aid in promoting labour, as well as in alleviating pain and other discomforts.

Points that facilitate Qi's descent and activate contractions are San Yin Jiao, Jian Jing and He Gu. Ci Liao and Yong Quan, along with Jian Jing are used to calm the mother. Note: these points should not be used during pregnancy.

SAN YIN JIAO

San Yin Jiao is located about three finger widths above the inside ankle on the shinbone (see illustration on page 97). It is tender to the touch. Apply strong pressure to this point with your thumb or index finger. Press towards the front of the mother's leg for thirty seconds, then stop for a thirty seconds. Repeat three or four times. Wait twenty minutes and apply pressure on the San Yin Jiao point on the opposite leg.

JIAN JING

To locate Jian Jing, imagine the midway point on an arc from the bony vertebra at the base of the neck (if you bend your head forward, it is generally the bone at the back of the neck that sticks out the most) to the shoulder joint. Jian Jing lies at the highest point of the muscle of the shoulder. Like San Yin Jiao, it too will feel tender to the touch, with a tingling, warm or numb sensation. Stimulating Jian Jing will stimulate the Uterus and is helpful during labour. Apply pressure with the thumbs and use the strength of the entire arm and not just the thumb. At the start of each contraction, press the point, or pressure can be continually applied and intensified with each contraction.

HE GU

He Gu is found between the first finger and the thumb in the V where the bones extending from the base of the index finger and thumb come together at the far end of the crease (see illustration below). Apply pressure to this point with the thumb for ten seconds, three times. Stimulation of this point can intensify contractions.

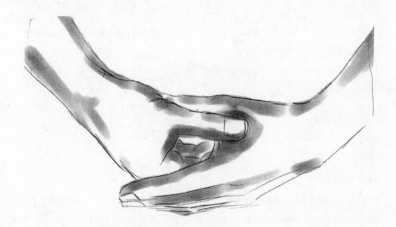

CI LIAO

To relax the mother and relieve pain, Ci Liao is used. This point lies halfway between the dimples that can be found above the buttock crease. It is approximately one of the mother's finger widths above the top of the crease of the buttocks and one of her thumb widths on each side of the spine. You will feel a slight depression when your finger is on this point. Apply pressure by placing the knuckles into the points and press down firmly (see illustration below). As the mother's labour progresses, apply pressure moving down the spine and moving hands closer together until the top of the buttock crease is reached. At this point the knuckles on each hand should be touching.

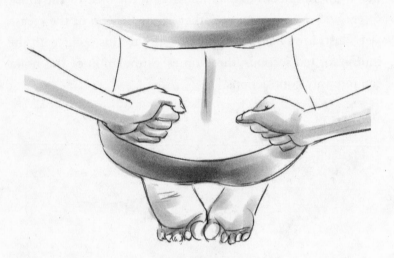

YONG QUAN

Yong Quan, also known as "Bubbling Spring," is another point used to help the mother relax. This point is found in the hollow that is formed in the top third of the sole of the foot when the toes are pushed towards the sole. Apply strong pressure in the hollow, pushing upwards and inwards towards the big toe (see illustration on page 96). This point can be used during all stages of labour.

SUMMARY

Healthy conception and pregnancy are intimately linked with the unobstructed and free flow of Heavenly Water. The Liver stores Blood, which is forwarded to the Uterus for discharge in menstruation or to nourish the fetus in utero. Factors that hamper the flow of Heavenly Water, then, will also affect the possibility of conception and proper fetal nourishment. The root cause of energetic imbalances that manifest as physical conditions in Heavenly Water, such as PMS and infertility, are the same emotional factors. So again, it is the free and appropriate expression of our feelings that is needed to conceive and to enjoy a healthy pregnancy. Working with our feelings, such as frustration and anger, will help to alleviate the physical condition that is blocking fertility and conception, or affecting health during pregnancy. If we can be as emotionally free as we are able, it will be that much easier to conceive and move through pregnancy into labour.

Having a baby brings tremendous changes—physically, emotionally and spiritually—within a relatively short period of time. Our ability to adjust and release firmly held identities and expectations plays a significant role in our ability to become pregnant and deliver a healthy newborn. In my practice, I have witnessed profound changes in my patients' capacities to conceive and bring a fetus full-term as they relinquish their beliefs about themselves. Their feelings and expectations of themselves while pregnant greatly influenced the kind of pregnancies they had.

Conversely, taking care of our physical conditions, such as premenstrual breast distension, may shift our feelings of anger or resentment. We cannot overlook that our physical health prior to conception is an important factor in a healthy pregnancy and birthing experience. Physical well-being depends on the balanced movement of Qi and Blood in our bodies. The free flow of Qi is none other than our emotional well-being, so even though we must address the physical manifestations of the imbalanced flow of Qi and Blood, we must also not lose sight of the root of the disharmony, our emotional disturbances. Our emotional distress and how it may further affect us as we go through specific physical changes are important to consider during our pregestational and gestational periods.

That which nourishes Kidney Essence will support conception and a healthy fetus. The health of our parents' Essence also contributed to the state of our constitution and our nature. If our parents' Essence was weak when we were conceived, then this would have been passed on to us. And we, in turn, pass our Essence on to our children. We can work to support our Kidney Essence by taking care not to consume it too rapidly or recklessly, or by preserving it through our Postnatal Essence. Essence will be less rapidly expended if we avoid overwork, frequent childbirth, chronic illness, sexual intercourse during menstruation, and if we are able to come to terms with our feelings.

We can also do much to conserve our Essence through our diet. If the amount of postnatal Essence extracted by the Spleen and Stomach through the food and drinks we consume is greater than what we expend daily, it will be stored in the Kidneys. This postnatal Essence is used before our prenatal Essence is tapped into. Therefore, eating foods and creating a conducive environment for the Spleen and Stomach to transform food into an abundance of postnatal Essence will assist in preserving and augmenting Kidney Essence.

The way we deal with our emotional and spiritual well-being, and the way we take care of our bodies through diet and lifestyle choices, all contribute to our capacity to allow the seed to naturally ripen into fruit, as well as allow the tree (the self) to grow along with it.

To help ourselves give birth, we may explore our fears of the unknown by understanding how we handle uncertainty. Our reaction to the unfamiliar is often related to our level of trust or mistrust in our inner selves. The beliefs we have about ourselves generally suppress our confidence in our bodies' innate knowledge of giving birth. This inner knowing, which we may call upon from deep within us, is an aspect of our collective wisdom.

By honouring ourselves and developing trust in our inner knowing, we can work with the uncertainty of labour and delivery. Childbirth is a time when the deep instinctual wisdom of the body is at work; if we distrust this, we may discover that we can't access the inner resources we need to deliver our babies. We can also respect the unknown of childbirth by increasing our knowledge of what will happen, practising visualization or meditation, or requesting the active participation of partners, family and friends. In whatever way we can, it is possible to begin to let go of our preconceived notions of childbirth and our fears of the uncertainty surrounding the birthing process, and trust the collective wisdom in our bodies. In this way, we open to connecting with the mystery of nature through giving birth, this natural process.

Part Six

GOLDEN MONTH

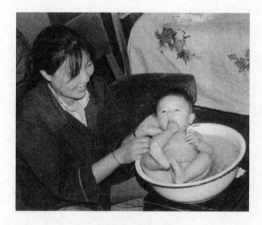

Me, bathing Zhao Zhao

CHAPTER FOURTEEN

Different Traditions

For some of us, vaginal delivery may not be an option. Zhao Zhao's delivery date was chosen and planned for February 22, 1984. My pregnancy was considered "high risk" as I had experienced a previous miscarriage and was considered old by Chinese standards, conceiving at the age of twenty-seven. My doctors thought that because I was "older," my bones would be less flexible, and they were also concerned that the placenta would adhere to the uterine wall, which could lead to postpartum hemorrhaging. Since the introduction of China's one-child policy in the late 1970s, special precautions were always taken to ensure the safety and health of an only child. Zhao Zhao was referred to as a "Treasure Baby" because of the possible complications, and my doctors strongly recommended that I have a Caesarean section.

When I went to the hospital on the predetermined delivery day, about twenty members of my family accompanied me: my husband, mother, father, mother-in-law, father-in-law, two sisters, brother, brothers-in-law, sisters-in-law, nieces and nephews. For Chinese families, a birth is an auspicious event, so it is common for this number of people to attend and bring food to nourish the mother.

When the time came for my Caesarean, I was given an epidural block, so that I wouldn't feel anything from the waist down. Acupuncture wasn't used because I was considered too weak at the time. I remember wanting to watch when the doctors made the incision, but my view was blocked with the white cotton sheet that was draped over the lower half of my body. I heard the metal sounds of the surgical instruments and requests for scissors. Prior to Zhao Zhao being lifted from me, I felt very weak and heard one of my colleagues say that my blood pressure had dropped. They quickly put an oxygen mask over my face. The next thing I remember was the sound of my baby crying! I would have to wait until the day after delivering him to hold him.

My son's official name is Jin Zhao, with Jin being his surname and Zhao being his first name. In China, the family name is always placed before the given name, showing the importance of the family over the individual. We chose the name Zhao because it means inner strength, something I continue to wish for my son as he lives his life. While Zhao is also my surname, it has a different character and meaning in Chinese. After his birth, we gave him the nickname of Zhao Zhao.

When I was in the recovery room, I felt the urge to move my bowels. I very much wanted to go to the toilet by myself. I slowly sat up, pulled out the catheter and put on my pants. I remember stepping on the floor and feeling as if there was nothing solid under my feet. It was like stepping on a thick carpet of cotton balls. With my second step, my body began to shake with the pain and my teeth started to chatter. Slowly I forced one foot in front of the other. In about twenty minutes, I had travelled only ten feet! Still, I managed to reach the toilet. After struggling with the pain of urinating and moving my bowels, I slowly rose. The moment I reached a standing position, I realized I had no strength left. I couldn't walk back to my bed. Fortunately, a nurse came into the room and quickly helped me. The medical staff was very concerned that I might have fainted from the pain and started to hemorrhage.

After delivery, women are often afraid to urinate or have a bowel movement because of fear of the pain. They may hold their urine, which can lead to urinary tract or bladder infections. I understood the importance of overcoming this initial fear and told myself that after this first time, going to the bathroom would not be as painful. To stimulate the flow of urine, a heated bag of salt can be used to warm up the abdominal area. Salt is used because it is associated with the Kidneys, which are related to the Bladder. Sometimes the woman's legs are spread open and warm water is splashed on the vulva. The sound of the water tinkling is thought to encourage and promote the free flow of urine.

When Zhao Zhao was brought to me, I did not have any milk in my breasts. Although it was painful to do, I began to use clean towels to massage my Uterus, as well as my breasts, to stimulate lactation. My mother brought sweet rice along with a dish of eggs and sugar water to encourage my breasts to lactate. Soon, I could feel milk filling my breasts. I wanted to breastfeed to bond with my baby, but also because breastfeeding promotes contractions in the Uterus, which can help prevent postpartum bleeding and assist the Uterus in resuming its normal tone and position.

I shared my postdelivery time with two other women who occupied the same room as myself. They were in their early twenties and I was considered the old one, at twenty-seven. We talked a great deal and shared many laughs. There was no privacy for any of us. The doctors and nurses examined and consulted with us in this room, and all our families crowded in and visited every day, bringing food to eat and share. My husband remained at the hospital for three consecutive days without leaving. He had brought a supply of fresh, clean pyjamas for me to change into, so I wouldn't have to lie in sweaty clothes and risk getting chilled. I did not bathe or shower or wash my hair. I cleansed my face and teeth with salt water and the nurses helped me to wash my vulva and vagina with a saline solution as well.

The nurses encouraged me to move and slowly begin to walk over the days following Zhao Zhao's birth. This is important after a C-section since gas tends to accumulate in the stomach. Moving also prevents the colon from collapsing and more deep-seated conditions such as a bowel obstruction.

When the time came for me to go home, my husband's company sent a car to pick us up. Since it was winter, I left the hospital wrapped head to toe, with the exception of my eyes. Great care was taken to ensure that Cold would not invade my body in the brief time I travelled in a wheelchair from the hospital into the awaiting car.

———

Unlike in the West, where women are often encouraged and applauded for leaving their beds and returning to their regular lives as quickly as possible after delivery, in China, the forty days following childbirth, referred to as "Golden Month," are given to the mother to rest, recover and regain her health. Much Blood is lost during and after childbirth, resulting in a Blood and Qi Deficiency, and a woman is therefore very susceptible to disease. Any illness she contracts during the postpartum period is believed to remain with her for the rest of her life. Moreover, any existing illness the mother has had prior to childbirth can be healed during Golden Month. In fact, on occasion, a doctor will advise a woman plagued with illnesses to become pregnant and use her Golden Month to restore her health. Such is the power to heal of this significant time. And this is why the month is called "Golden."

During Golden Month, a woman makes every effort to build her Blood and support the restoration of her Kidney strength and energy. Childbirth, especially frequent childbirth, can dramatically deplete Essence, or Jing, leading to mental and physical degeneration and reducing one's lifespan. In order to support her Kidneys and preserve her Essence, she takes time away from ordinary life to avoid excessive stress, emotional disturbances, overwork and fatigue, and she takes great care to eat well. In this she is supported by family and friends. If there is no family to help, husbands often hire women to assist the new mother. Proper treatment during this month will prevent future ill health, which may cost the family a great deal more.

In Canada, I once visited one of my patients in the hospital who had just given birth to her son. I remember my shock in arriving the evening of her delivery to find a room full of flowers but devoid of people. Candy was in great pain, having undergone a Caesarean section, and her newborn was crying in the bassinet by her bed. Her lips were dry, her face was pale and no one was there to help her. I quickly asked her if she was hungry, and she said she was starving. I asked my partner to run down to Chinatown and bring her back some congee, or rice porridge, to eat. In the meantime, I helped Candy drink some fluids and changed her son's diapers.

This was such a different experience than what I was accustomed to. I really felt a cultural divide in that moment. As I described earlier, in China, childbirth is a family affair and is honoured as a special time when family and friends welcome the baby and give the mother the special attention needed to regain her health. There is a sense of connection between the generations and a continuation of the ancestral lineage, a sense that childbirth is a collective and collaborative life event.

In the West, there is often an abundance of beautiful flowers after childbirth, but there's not much help from family members. They generally don't stay in the hospital with the mother, thinking she needs rest. The responsibility for her physical needs are relegated to the hospital and its staff. Though flowers are beautiful and symbolic in meaning, they offer no support in restoring a woman's energy and health at a critical time. After Zhao Zhao was born, even if I rested, my family remained. The support they offered by their presence was very important to me and helped me get through those first days, then weeks, with love, care and physical help. Perhaps this family involvement in China is one of the reasons that there is a much lower incidence of postpartum depression as compared to the West. To this day, whenever a friend or patient has given birth, I always cook a pot of soup to give to the mother, and I take this to her, along with flowers, with the hope that it will start her off on a Golden Month of healing and prevention.

Delivering a baby results in a loss of Yang, which is used to discharge the baby from the Uterus. As a result, a woman is in a state of Cold and is extremely susceptible to Cold penetrating and lodging in the body. Therefore, she should abstain from bathing, washing her hair, lifting heavy items, exposing herself to cold water or cold temperatures or wind, swimming, eating cold foods (such as salads or uncooked foods), drinking cold fluids, sexual intercourse and excessive exercise. If a mother does not observe these practices, she will be subject to pain, aches, arthritis and other illnesses in the future.

To regain Yang, or Heat, and restore energy and balance to her system, a new mother must eat Yang foods that are warming in nature, such as lamb and other red meats, red kidney beans and lentils. Blood must be built up for a woman to be restored to full health, and a simple dish like the egg soup I mentioned in Chapter Three (see recipe on page 56) is effective in enhancing Blood.

After I was born in May 1956, my mother stayed in the hospital for six days. When she was ready to leave, she covered her head, dressed warmly and walked home with my aunt, who carried me. When my mother arrived at our apartment, the room was cold, since there was no heating in the building. She remembers feeling the cold in her body as she lay on her bed. Cooking an egg was not an easy thing for my mother to do. At the time of my birth, apartments in China did not have kitchens. People ate communally in cafeterias at their places of

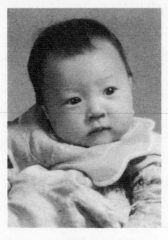

Me, as an infant

employment and were at the mercy of whatever the cook decided to put on the menu. Fortunately, the food served in the cafeteria was fresh and of very good quality. Many choices of vegetables that were not overcooked and a variety of meats were offered daily. Eggs, however, were not abundant, and if served at the cafeteria, would not be prepared with raw cane sugar. Somehow my grandmother managed to get a precious egg, and using alcohol as fuel and a can as a pot, cooked egg soup for my mother to eat.

The importance of these self-care practices is ingrained in every Chinese woman from childhood, and is passed on from one generation to the next. Though my mother was well aware of them, she unfortunately ended up lifting during her Golden Month and also put her hands in cold water to wash clothes. Because the temperature in our home was cool during the latter part of May, she often felt chilly. Consequently, she developed wrist pain and headaches that she had never experienced prior to my birth, and these conditions have remained with her till the present.

MY GOLDEN MONTH

When I returned home after the birth of Zhao Zhao, my mother came to cook and support me every day from seven in the morning until two in the afternoon. Her caring was so complete and devoted, I felt totally nurtured and loved. From two to nine in the evening, my mother-in-law took over. My husband, too, spent at least an hour every day taking care of me, and I also had a nanny whose sole responsibility was to wash diapers and clothes and look after Zhao Zhao when I was resting. We considered this help an investment in my current recovery and future health.

During Golden Month, I remained at home and kept my head, arms, legs and body covered. Zhao Zhao and I did not go outdoors at all. A newborn infant, like his mother, is considered vulnerable to external causes of disharmony. I sweated continually during the days following the delivery, which is quite common and a result of Blood and Qi Deficiency. Generally, if sweating occurs during the night, this is due to Yin or Blood Deficiency, and if sweating occurs during the day, it is a result of a Qi insufficiency. Perspiring is not considered a problem unless it is profuse and continues over a prolonged period of time. If this happens, avoid eating cold, raw and uncooked foods and cold drinks, keep away from cold, damp rooms, keep your body and head covered and eat Blood-enhancing foods such as dates, raisins, eggs, spinach, liver, sweet black rice and pork. In enriching Blood, both Qi and Essence are also nourished.

In spite of all the perspiration, I did not bathe or shower, or wash my hair. Instead, I had frequent sponge baths with ginger water, which is made by boiling fresh ginger in a pot of water. I loved the fragrance of the ginger that permeated my skin and clothes, and even though I did not completely submerge my body or use soap, I felt clean and refreshed. Ginger's heating properties warm the body when it is Qi and Blood deficient.

Every day, my husband or mother would give me a ginger treatment to alleviate the headaches I had suffered from prior to my pregnancy. They would wrap a whole, fresh ginger root between green cabbage leaves and roast it for an hour in the oven. The cooked ginger would then be sliced and, while still warm, placed on my temples, between my eyebrows and on the crown of my head. They would then wrap my head with a cloth to hold the ginger in place. To this day, I have never experienced a recurrence of headaches.

My husband would also place ginger on my back in the area of my Kidneys and tie surgical cloth around it to hold the ginger in place. This was to support the Kidney Organ system, clear Cold and reduce back pain.

In addition to the ginger treatment, my husband would apply castor oil to my abdomen and massage my Uterus. After the massage, he would cover this area with surgical cloth and tightly wrap my body. This was to tighten the muscles in my abdomen, make my skin firm and taut, and help my Uterus regain its normal tone and strength.

Many friends visited me during this time. My friends who were TCM doctors would give me acupuncture treatments to unblock my Kidney channels and promote and enhance the flow of depleted energy. Others would bring gifts—generally of food—and in keeping with tradition, I would offer them sweet foods, such as a dish of eggs and cane sugar, or rice wine. This gesture symbolized a sharing of my happiness with them.

Aside from visiting with friends and family, I rested. I wasn't supposed to strain my eyes by reading or watching television. For the first week, I was able to adhere to these practices, but after a while I found myself reading a bit. I was careful not to read too much, because I could feel my eyes easily tiring. After a couple of weeks, I started to watch the occasional television program.

My days revolved around my intake of food. I ate many small meals throughout the day to strengthen my Spleen Qi, which in turn would further nourish and replenish my Kidney Essence. Eating frequent, small meals instead of one or two large ones doesn't overtax the Spleen system. To build Spleen Qi and enrich Blood, I would eat egg soup for breakfast every day. Most of the typical problems that arise after childbirth are associated with the loss of Blood. Hair loss, for example, is closely related to Blood loss, as is postpartum depression. This is because a tremendous loss of Blood can lead to insufficient Blood in the Heart, which transforms food Essence into Blood and circulates it. The Spirit, or Shen, resides in the Heart, so insufficient Blood in this Organ system may cause a new mother to feel lethargic, unable to sleep, unable to bond with her baby, unrelenting despair, worthlessness, sadness, anxiety, apathy or feeling separate from reality.

Thus, it is important to eat foods that nourish the Blood and support the Heart, Kidneys, Liver and Spleen—the Organs that are vital to the production and movement of Blood. Some of the foods that are traditionally eaten to support these Organ systems are chicken, fish, green leafy vegetables, eggs, raisins, sweet rice and dried longan fruit.

About one hour after breakfast, I would eat an herbal chicken soup that contained *Yimu Cao*, commonly known as motherwort, to help the Uterus regain its normal size and tone, and prevent excessive bleeding related to a Deficiency in the Uterus. Chicken soup provides the warmth needed to increase Yang energy and to dispel the Cold state of the body, and nourish Blood. Every day I ate soup made from the stock of one chicken. Over seven days, I ate the equivalent stock and meat of seven chickens! Some days, the chicken soup would contain dried longan fruit, which builds Blood by nourishing the Heart Organ system. Its sweet taste also assists the Spleen in recovering and assimilating the nutrients in the soup.

Herbal Chicken Soup

1	4-pound chicken
12 cups	cold water
60 grams	*Yimu Cao* (motherwort)
40 grams	*Dong Quai* (angelica)

1. Place chicken in a large pot and add cold water. Bring to a boil, reduce heat and simmer for 2 hours. Drink the broth and eat the cooked chicken throughout the day.

I ate chicken soup several times a day. My mother encouraged me to use my hands when I ate the chicken so that the fat would lubricate my skin. The soup also helped replenish the fluid that I lost through sweating and the loss of Blood. Moreover, soups and other liquids help to counter constipation if you are breastfeeding and not drinking lots of fluids.

Bone soups, which contain marrow, are beneficial in nourishing Blood, Essence and the Kidneys. These soups also help prevent the joint pain that is common after childbirth. (See a recipe for bone soup on page 186.) Another way to avoid pain in the joints is to keep warm and minimize exposure to cold temperatures and drafts.

In addition to soup, I ate lightly cooked vegetables one or two times a day and cooked fruit. I never ate them raw, since raw foods are more difficult for the already weakened Spleen and Stomach to digest. It is also said that eating cold foods during Golden Month will make the mother's teeth sensitive for the remainder of her life.

In order to produce milk, a woman needs adequate Blood and Qi. The flow of milk can be effectively stimulated by eating milk-promoting foods, the most traditional of which is pork hock boiled in black vinegar and ginger, which nourishes Blood and Qi and warms the body. During my mother's Golden Month, my grandmother, with very limited resources, made sure to cook a pork hock for her on a makeshift stove. Papaya and peanuts are two other foods that help stimulate lactation.

Pork Hock

1	pork hock
5 cups	black vinegar (available in Asian grocery stores)
$1/4$ pound	fresh, sliced ginger root

1. Wash the pork hock with cold water. Place pork hock in a large pot and add enough cold water to cover. Bring to a boil, reduce heat and simmer for 10 minutes.

2. Drain the pork hock, and rinse it with cold water. Place the pork hock back in the pot and add the black vinegar and sliced ginger. Bring to a boil, reduce heat and simmer for 1 hour. Drain pork hock and slice before serving.

If you are breastfeeding, avoid spicy, overly rich and greasy dishes, and foods that are not easily digested, such as raw foods and legumes. Sometimes we do not express much or any milk even though we produce a sufficient volume. This is generally caused by Liver Qi Stagnation in the Meridians that pass through the breasts, since Qi is required to express milk. Whatever we can do to become aware of any anger, resentment or frustration we may feel will help to encourage lactation, given that the Liver system is so intertwined with our emotional well-being. The free flow of emotions is directly related to the free flow of Liver Qi and the free movement of breast milk.

When feeding your baby, try to empty your breasts of all the milk. Squeeze or pump out as much as you can if your baby doesn't drink it or if you still feel heaviness in your breasts. This will prevent milk from stagnating and will encourage its ongoing production. If your glands become clogged, apply hot, wet towels to your breasts to help open the glands. If your doctor has diagnosed an infection in your glands, apply cold, wet towels to your breasts. Also, drink lots of soup and warm liquids.

During the second half of my Golden Month, I started to do very gentle stretching to prevent Qi and Blood from stagnating. Try the simple exercises suggested on the next page—

remember to start slowly and be gentle. It is not advisable to engage in excessive physical exertion, as it can weaken the Spleen and Kidneys.

- Lie on your back with legs straight, arms at sides. Slowly inhale and pull your navel towards your back, pressing your back to the floor. Hold this position and then relax. This exercise can also be done while you're standing or sitting.
- Lie on your back with knees bent and feet flat on the floor. Tighten the muscles of your vagina as if you were trying to stop the flow of urine. If you are not sure you are working with the right muscle, check by placing a finger in your vagina. Try tightening the muscle around it. If you feel pressure around your finger, you will know you are using the right muscle. Hold for a count of five, then release.
- Lie on your back with your knees bent and your arms at your sides. Tighten your stomach, pulling your navel towards your back and lift one leg towards your chest with the knee bent. Exhale as you slowly straighten your leg so it is parallel with the floor but not touching the floor. Gently return to your starting position. Repeat with the other leg.
- Try a walking meditation. Like other forms of meditation, walking can be relaxing as well as a way to develop awareness and mindfulness in the moment. This slow and natural walk is based on paying attention to each foot as it makes contact with the floor. Stand tall, and allow the Qi to move through to your arms

and legs. Relax your shoulders, making sure that they are not up around your ears. Keep your breathing slow and regular. Try to breathe into your abdomen, so that with each in-breath, your stomach expands slightly and with each out-breath, it contracts. Soften your stomach. Keep your eyes lowered and focused a few feet ahead. If your mind wanders, simply take note of where it went and return your attention back to each foot touching the floor. Pay attention as you lift your foot, move it forward, then place it back on the floor. Continue for as long as you feel comfortable. Walking meditation, with its calming benefits and the emergence of awareness, can help you deal with the stresses and changes that accompany giving birth.

The end of Golden Month is celebrated with a ritual bath containing a mixture of herbs prescribed by a TCM practitioner, which signifies the close of the "official" period of resting and restoration for the mother, and marks her return to regular life. The herbs are therapeutic in removing Damp from the mother's muscles and joints, and assure a pain- and ache-free future.

It had been over a month since I had washed my hair and soaked my body in water. It was so wonderful to sit in the bath and allow the water to wash over me, inhaling the smell of the fragrant herbs. I felt rejuvenated and renewed. The herbal bath was a beautifully symbolic way to begin life in the world afresh as a mother.

(I think it is important to note here that after I miscarried my first baby, I carried out the same practices that I have outlined here for about fifteen days—a "small Golden Month." The preventative measures help prevent future health problems and complications.)

When I emerged from Golden Month, my nails were strong, my skin was glowing and my hair was rich in colour. I was well-rested, and nourished physically as well as emotionally and spiritually. I felt able to return to work and, most importantly, to ease into and fulfill my role as a mother. I cannot stress how crucial this time is for a woman's well-being and health. Today, new mothers often visit my clinic, excited to show me their week-old infants. When I see them, I cringe. I want to say to them, "Please go home and rest for one month. Your body is very vulnerable. You're putting yourself at risk for developing problems that will afflict you in the future. Your baby also isn't strong and you're putting her in a compromising position needlessly. Take this time to regain your health and heal the illnesses that have bothered you. It is only one month out of your life, but it has the power to impact your and your baby's health positively or negatively for the rest of your lives."

Perhaps some of you who are reading this book will find the practices of Golden Month reminiscent of what your grandmothers or great-grandmothers taught. They are really not too foreign. It is my hope that you will consider following, or even passing along, some of these self-care measures. They are based on millennia of life experience in China.

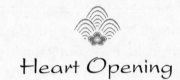

CHAPTER FIFTEEN

Heart Opening

There is an adage in China that says, "Only when you have a child, will you know how much your parents have given to you." Once I had Zhao Zhao, all the complaints and disagreements I had with my parents seemed so trivial. I had a new appreciation of what they had gone through in having me. I came to see my parents in a new light. Having personally experienced childbirth, I now shared a similar understanding of the miracle of birth, and in this way, was connected to them differently from before. New feelings of gratitude for them rose inside of me.

During Golden Month, my feelings of responsibility for my son, this vulnerable, helpless life, really began to sink in. For the first while, I felt as though it was all a dream. Even though I had carried Zhao Zhao inside of me, I was amazed that this tiny human being had come out of my body. Where had he come from? How had this happened?

Sometimes I would look at him and find him so foreign. I

would pick up his little hands and examine his fingers and nails, I would look at his nose and into his eyes, and it was like seeing fingers and nails, and a nose and eyes for the first time. And, in some ways, I *was* giving birth to a new way of seeing this perfect, miniature human being.

I would gently wash Zhao Zhao's body and feel a sense of total focus and commitment to cleaning him. It was as if nothing else mattered but to cleanse and nurture his tiny arms and hands, legs and feet, torso and head. I realized in those moments that there was nothing I expected from him. There was nothing he had to give me. His presence was all that mattered. It was of no consequence what he did; he was never a bother or irritation. Every one of his actions and sounds was a new and profound experience for me.

I love to sleep and can be grouchy and ill-tempered if I am disturbed. In the past, my irritation spared no one. Even my dear grandmother, who took such tender care of me, would see my grumpiness if she inadvertently woke me from a deep sleep. With Zhao Zhao, there was a radical shift. With the first sound from his throat, I would be awake, without a trace of ill feeling. My only concern was his well-being. I would often say, "I'm not afraid of the sky, I'm not afraid of the earth. The only thing I'm afraid of is of Zhao Zhao getting sick."

Zhao Zhao opened my heart to giving unconditional love. In my life, I had received absolute love from my parents, my grandmother and my family. But when Zhao Zhao was born, it was like I finally truly knew what love was. I experienced a sense of total, abiding love for him that didn't ask anything in return. My unconditional love for him connected me with my mother. I felt my mother's love anew and had a deeper understanding of her feelings for me, for all her children. And I also felt the love of all mothers for their children. Perhaps not every new mother feels what I did, but for me, childbirth brought me out of myself and into profound connection with my son, my mother and other human beings.

It seems to me that life before Zhao Zhao was a lot about me, my goals, dreams, plans, wants and needs. Not that I didn't take others into consideration, but I realized that I most often had an expectation of the other person that was connected to what *I* wanted or needed or desired. With Zhao Zhao, all of that fell away. I seemed to forget about my ego in my love for him, and in doing so, I was able to bring more heart and feeling to my work as a doctor. Though I had always been an attentive physician, I realized I had been there for my patients with my head only. I had adopted an intellectual approach to working with patients, not an emotional one. Allowing myself to surrender to the intense feelings that arose in giving birth to my son helped me connect with others on a deeper level, and I was able to integrate this into my work, bringing greater compassion, understanding, care and patience to others.

There was once a great Buddhist master who asked three of his students to explain apples to him. As he placed an apple on the table, he said to them, "Whoever can best tell me about apples will get to go on a retreat with me." One student spoke of the origin of apples and how they were introduced into their country. The second student talked of the different uses of apples in making desserts, ciders and sauces. The third student was silent as he pulled a small knife from his pocket. He proceeded to cut a slice off the apple and put it the master's mouth. Then he gently pushed the master's jaw up so that he would bite the apple. "Yes, this is it," said the master to the third student. "We cannot use words to describe an apple. It must be experienced by the tongue, teeth and mouth. The way to truly know an apple is to keep your mouth shut." Like knowing about an apple, the only way to know our deep feelings is not through our minds and our conceptual thoughts, but through experiencing them with our hearts.

Motherhood has the most incredible possibilities for enhancing all aspects of our lives. Sometimes this happens because we are able to surrender and trust in the process. I never planned or thought that having Zhao Zhao would change my ideas and identity so dramatically; or maybe on an unconscious level I did. Maybe this is what we all fear in becoming pregnant and giving birth: a loss of or change in identity or relationship with ourselves and others, a shift from the known or familiar to the unknown. I believe that all of our concepts and thoughts about the way things "should be" are shattered or displaced in the process of childbirth. Birthing doesn't allow for control. We give birth and experience an ultimate letting go, a trusting in a process much larger than we have the capacity to govern: the miracle of life. When we can surrender our small, limited ideas of what should happen, our expectations, or who we should be, then there is an opening to a greater awareness that is powerfully spiritual in its interconnectedness to something larger than ourselves.

SUMMARY

Golden Month is the special time following childbirth when a mother rests, restores and recovers her energy. With Chinese medicine's focus on prevention, Golden Month is a culturally recognized time to rebuild strength and fortify the body, and thereby guard against potential disease in the future. It is said that if a new mother does not adhere to the prescribed practices, illnesses will result that will afflict her for the duration of her life. As well, Golden Month is a period of healing. Existing illnesses may be eliminated or greatly alleviated with proper care.

The self-care measures during Golden Month are primarily focused on restoring the body's balance after an excessive loss of Qi and Blood during childbirth. With the discharge of Blood, there is also a loss of Essence. A woman can conserve and build her Essence, Qi and Blood by resting, not becoming fatigued, maintaining emotional balance, eating Blood-enriching foods and avoiding external conditions, such as Cold, that may compromise the mother's weakened condition. Following these practices requires the support of family and friends in looking after the mother's special needs and taking care of the baby so that the mother is able to rest.

Golden Month gives a mother the opportunity to regain her strength and energy before moving fully into her role as mother. Observing a period during which we acknowledge the radical changes that have occurred and the impact this has on our lives is one way to give love and nourishment, which we are generally so willing to give to others, to ourselves. It allows us the space to experience the connection between our physical, emotional and spiritual levels of well-being.

There is a humbleness that comes with realizing the incredible miracle of life developing and being birthed without our direction or intervention. The growth and development of Zhao Zhao inside me was guided by an inner wisdom that is not intellectual or conceptual. It is something that resides within every woman. With this awareness is a wonderful connectedness to others. And Golden Month brings another connection: it is a tradition that is handed down from one generation to the next, linking my mother to me, and me to my grandmother, one mother to the next, through the shared experience of birthing a baby. All people who are living and have lived have been born from women. It is a huge task we have taken on. I feel that Golden Month is one way for us to acknowledge and respect the significance of this work, to foster self-empowerment, and to honour the miracle of creation and the innate collective wisdom within us.

Part Seven

SECOND SPRING

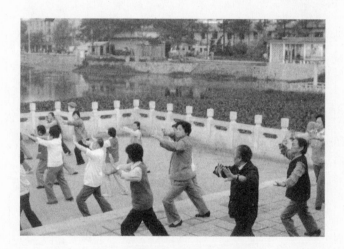

Practising Tai Chi in Kunming

CHAPTER SIXTEEN

Moving into Wholeness

In Traditional Chinese Medicine, the stage in a woman's life following the cessation of the flow of Heavenly Water is referred to as "Second Spring" to represent a renewal of energy and opportunities. In the West, the transition is known as menopause, a term derived from Greek that means the stopping of the monthly period. However, the association of menopause with an abrupt absence of periods is a limited view of this complex transition. Our passage to Second Spring takes place over a number of years and involves an intricate and complicated series of changes that is not restricted to our periods or the physical realm. For a small percentage of us, our periods will stop suddenly, while most of us will undergo irregularity in our cycles for two to five years before the permanent loss of our menstrual cycle. Some of us will notice changes a decade prior to the beginning of Second Spring. Generally, a woman is said to be menopausal when there has been a complete cessation of menstruation for six to twelve months after the age of forty-five. According to Western medicine, this is due to decreased production of hormones in midlife. The number of ovarian follicles, which are responsible for our reproductive force, decreases from approximately 600,000 at birth to 300,000 at the onset of menses, to about 10,000 when our periods stop. Thus, menopause is a progression that begins at birth.

According to the *Nei Jing*, Second Spring is the third important phase in a woman's reproductive life, following Heavenly Water and childbirth. As we know, a woman's life evolves in seven-year cycles, and after our Heavenly Water begins to flow at the age of fourteen, we reach our peak time of development from age twenty-one to twenty-eight. When we reach thirty-five (seven times five), our Spleen starts to slow down, and the production of Blood, Qi and postnatal Essence decreases. Because muscles are also governed by the Spleen, as it weakens, muscles start to slacken and wrinkles form. By the age of forty-nine (seven times seven) we have less Blood, Qi and postnatal Essence and must use more of our stored prenatal Essence. With less Blood produced, the Penetrating Vessel, which carries Blood to the Uterus, will not be full, and as a consequence, the Uterus will not overflow with its excess. Our Heavenly Water will diminish and eventually cease. In an effort to conserve our Essence as much as possible, the wisdom of our bodies stops the monthly discharge of Blood. It is interesting that the cessation of our periods is generally perceived as the advancement of aging, when it is, in fact, our bodies' natural effort to slow down this process and bring new balance to our advancing years.

Since Blood and Essence are no longer being lost on a

monthly basis, the energy that had been used to ensure an adequate supply of Blood is freed up for us to do with as we choose. As a result, we feel rejuvenated and experience an awakening of new potential—Second Spring. The transition marks a change in Yin relative to Yang energy, since less Blood, which is Yin, is produced. Traditionally, in our premenopausal years, we are focused on relationships, careers, creating a family and home. Our attention is often on nurturing and caring for others. Women who have careers outside the home are, typically, still responsible for looking after the children and the household. Often our self-esteem and identities have been defined and also compromised by our relationships. We are a wife of so-and-so, or the mother of, or the daughter of. Even though we may have a career, the cultural pressures to be identified in relationship, traditionally with a man, are very strong.

In many cases, then, being in the world comes later for women, as we develop an independent sense of self. Our power and achievements very often manifest at mid-life and beyond. This is a manifestation of our more apparent Yang energy. We become more passionate about our beliefs. We're able to express our anger. We are more apt to stand up for ourselves. There is a well-known Chinese saying: "Women in their thirties are wolves; in their forties, tigers, and their fifties, dragons."

DIANE

For most of her adult life, Diane could safely say that she was most confident in how to love a man and make him happy. She wasn't able to exercise her will in the world and develop a career or deal with conflict, but she said she was a nice,

sweet woman who could soothe and care for others, especially men. Her Yin side was developed, but she was like a
child in her Yang energy. She says, "I couldn't grab hold of a
goal and move through it. I hadn't fully completed the stages
of autonomy that I needed to function in the world. But I felt
confident in my ability to support a man's goals and make life
work for him."

When Diane was forty-eight years old, her second husband left her. Within six months, she met Paul, a man to fulfill her sense of worth and purpose. In him, she found the
support, power and strength that she lacked, and fell in love
with him. Five years later, however, Paul had a stroke. He suffered significant capacity and memory loss and was no longer
able to complete daily tasks. While he had been a professional
engineer, he now could not remember how to turn on a radio
or make a cup of tea. Suddenly Diane had to assume responsibility for the structure of their lives. The qualities she needed
from Paul weren't there, and she felt overwhelmed.

Three years after his stroke, Paul had a recurrence of the
prostate cancer he'd had when he was younger. The cancer
had metastasized and he required radiation for pain in his hip.
His health rapidly declined. Suffering from a form of demen-
tia, Paul would be angry, paranoid and judgmental at times.
Diane discovered that if she got angry back at him for his rage,
in the next moment he might ask, "What's for lunch?" She
says, "Initially I was surprised to find out that he hadn't gone
away. He was still here." When Paul became paranoid and
thought people were trying to murder him, Diane would
explain that there were no people or she would try to distract
him. Still, he would insist they were coming to the apartment.

One day, Diane looked at him during one of these moments and realized how terrified he really was. Understanding his sheer terror in a new way, she says, "A power rose in me. I said to Paul, 'There's no one coming through this door. I'll hurt them and kill them. The power of hell will not come through this door.'" Paul looked at her and said, "Oh, OK." And that was the end of his paranoia. Diane was able to access her power to make Paul feel safe.

Paul died about a year after the return of his cancer, a few years after his stroke and eight years after Diane and he had met. She says, "I am coming out of this with intactness and wholeness, with a sense of fullness and emptiness, finding a sense of full selfness and emptiness at the same time." Today, at fifty-six, Diane says that in journeying towards wholeness, "It is important to live through things and test our beliefs and who we are. And this takes time."

For many of us, uncovering our sense of self may require waiting until the rising of our Yang energy in our Second Spring. We are now able to use the experience and knowledge gained in our lives to express ourselves authentically, renewed in a new stage of our evolution. In this way, we may feel as though Second Spring is gifting us with a new opportunity.

The process of aging is really a journey towards wholeness, where all aspects of our being, our Jing, or Essence, Qi and Shen—the Three Treasures—are cultivated and balanced to become harmoniously engaged. In the first half of our lives, Jing, the physicality of our bodies, and Qi, our feelings for others and ourselves, seem to occupy most of our attention. But as Blood stops flowing to our Uterus, it is now free to be sent to our Heart. Here it nourishes Shen, which is the inner spirit of our selves. For this reason, we may feel a desire to fulfill our spiritual and higher needs. Our interest tends to shift from the material to the satisfaction and quality of our lives, the realm of Shen, which is greatly affected by our cognitive mind, emotions and cumulative life experiences. Often we need to clarify our identities, who we are, and strengthen our sense of self. Sometimes we embark on a search of meaning and purpose. Maybe we're looking for peace, or perhaps it's authentic love we're seeking. The movement towards meeting our spiritual and higher needs will be as individual as each of us is. We may write the story of our lives, move to the country, let go of a long-held grudge, deepen an existing relationship, join a meditation or prayer group, return to school, start volunteering, do something we've always dreamed of doing or stop doing something we've always been doing. We may begin to consider our lives according to the years we have left instead of the years we've lived; what we want to do instead of focusing on what we've done.

To bring Shen into harmony is to reflect inward on our journey. Sometimes it is the accumulation of life experiences that catapults us into a spiritual search. Perhaps the changes or the losses we face in our menopausal years and thereafter nudge us or hurl us towards exploring what we need spiritually.

I was reintroduced to Buddhism in my late thirties by a former patient of mine, who taught me how to meditate. My grandmother had been Buddhist, and I remember frequently going with her to the market to buy live fish for the Buddhist ceremony of releasing fish and turtles. This ceremony is a symbolic gesture of setting ourselves free from our own desires. Freed, we can concentrate our minds on helping other living beings and ultimately attain enlightenment. In Buddhism, enlightenment is a state of pure and unqualified knowledge and intuitive insight, in which things are seen as they truly are. The ceremony is also a demonstration of one's compassion for all living creatures. All life has the capacity for higher consciousness; therefore no sentient life should be impeded, hindered or harmed in their efforts. By releasing fish, Buddhists manifest their compassion for all living beings on a physical as well as symbolic level.

After my grandmother had bought the fish, we would go to the edge of the canal and she would release the fish into the water. I watched this and felt it would be wonderful to be a fish or a bird, because they have great freedom. Other than this ceremony, my memories of Buddhism in China are of people going to the temple and praying. I heard prayers for more money, better health and improved grades, and thought, "Why doesn't that person just work harder to get more money, or take better care of their health, or study harder?" Buddhism seemed steeped in superstition and was not an active aspect of my life.

Being able to reconnect with Buddhism in Canada allowed me to rediscover and appreciate this ancient belief system anew. Though Traditional Chinese Medicine has its origins in Taoism, Confucianism and Buddhism, it is not necessary to practise or understand these philosophies and religions in order to benefit from Chinese medicine. But Buddhism has helped me reconnect with spirituality and myself in a new way and has greatly opened me up to compassion for myself and for others. Belief systems may provide us with insights and understanding as we try to find a way to satisfy our spiritual needs in Second Spring. As we search, they may help us to feel harmonious and peaceful, especially as we face the changes, stresses, joys and sorrows of aging.

The transition to Second Spring is a time fraught with mixed feelings, reactions and experiences that are unique to each of us. We may view it as the entry into owning the wisdom we've gathered in our lives. Conversely, some may approach this transition with fear, afraid of aging. Others may feel that we've finally mastered a sense of influence over our relationships, finances and work. Or we may regret that we haven't accomplished what we had hoped to by this point in our lives. We might feel saddened at the loss of our fertility or elated at being freed from the worries of contraception. We may experience uncertainty and confusion, wondering, "Who will need me or want me now?" Or we may feel relief in realizing that what others think of us doesn't hold as much sway as it used to. How we think about this life stage is a result of our cultural, societal and personal experiences, and plays a critical role in how we are able to embrace, move through and accept this natural life phase.

Our attitudes have as much influence on how we experience the transition as our biochemistry does. As women, it is not part of our biological makeup to value a specific ideal body shape or role or age. These are culturally determined. The way our society and popular media define aging women affects how we, as aging women, view ourselves. Since our perceptions shape our emotions, they affect our psychological, physiological and spiritual well-being. It is helpful, then, to be aware of our culture-specific definitions of menopausal women and aging. Before exploring our Western attitudes, I would like to share my perceptions and feelings around the transition into Second Spring as a woman born and raised in China. My experiences of the journey from my reproductive to nonreproductive years are deeply coloured by my cultural background and my direct experience of, and with, it.

In Chinese culture, there is a sense of looking forward to old age, since the elderly are revered and given special respect. Confucius (551–479 BCE) was the founder of the social ethics and moral teachings that largely impact Chinese life and thought. He taught that there will be peace and happiness for all people when we treat not only our own parents as our parents, not only our own children as our children, when the sick are taken care of, when people who are able are fully employed, when the young are provided with a nurturing upbringing and when the elderly have a meaningful existence until they die. These basic conditions for harmony are based on love and the importance of relationships.

Embedded in these teachings of relationships is great esteem for age. It is thought that with age comes wisdom. In China, people generally do not start to celebrate birthdays until after their sixtieth year. This is considered an important milestone, an age to be proud of. It is an opportunity for children, family members and friends to acknowledge their elders and show respect and express their gratitude for what they have done and given in their lives. The older one is, the greater the cause for celebration. Seniors are respected and revered for their collected and collective wisdom.

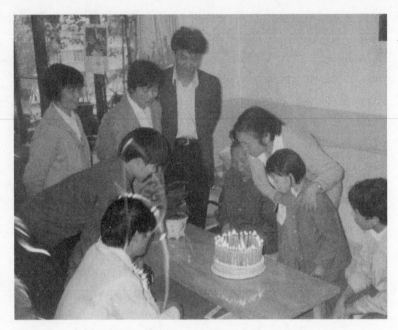

My grandmother's eightieth birthday party

This perspective is very different from Western society's, where youthfulness is worshipped, and the aged are marginalized, negatively stereotyped or disregarded altogether. How often have we seen older women depicted as silly or forgetful, nonsexual or retiring? Perhaps the Western emphasis on individualism and independence is a factor in the loss of value of the aged. The desire to retain our self-sufficiency is in danger as we become vulnerable to the frailties of aging, or as we lose our ability to economically support ourselves. If we become dependent on others, we are no longer free agents. We view ourselves and are viewed by others as burdens. If we are able to take care of ourselves, we often do it apart from our families, since generally, extended-family living is not part of North

American culture. To live on one's own as an elderly person is seen as a positive sign of independence. But it may also involve a loss of intimate relationships with loved ones and a further distancing of one's self from others.

In China, the family is the primary source of physical, economic and emotional care for older people. The responsibility to support elderly family members is a deeply held cultural tradition and obligation. Most older people live in extended households of several generations and maintain an important role in the family. They have a respected place and a sense of purpose.

In the West there is a tendency to define value by what we do. So often I have been in social gatherings where one of the most common conversational gambits is: "What do you do?" If we retire or are no longer at the peak of our careers, our sense of worth may be compromised. As well, we may associate our "productive" years with our fertility. With the signs of menopause, we may feel that our worth as defined by our ability to procreate is threatened and thereby experience a profound feeling of "emptiness" or "incompleteness." We may feel we are no longer a productive and vital part of society. With a decline of function comes a negative change of attitudes directly associated with cultural norms and misnomers.

As I enter my menopausal years, I have reflected on my attitudes towards aging, as a woman born in China, who now lives in Canada. In the West we are bombarded by messages that promote physical attractiveness, vitality and youth. These are the socially acceptable and valued qualities as defined by the culture, and we often feel pressured to subscribe to them, shaping ourselves literally and metaphorically to fit the ideal. As we age, it becomes increasingly more difficult to meet the standards that the West has adopted and promoted, and this can affect how we feel about and value ourselves. As I mentioned in Part Two, "Heavenly Water," there was a time when I was much more vulnerable to these messages, but as I grow older I feel more grounded in who I am and have greater acceptance of myself. This is not to say that I welcome grey hair, facial wrinkles, loss of memory or reading glasses, but I see them as natural aspects of the evolution of life, from birth to death.

We may find it difficult to accept the inevitabilities and unknown aspects of aging and the changes it brings. We may feel we are losing our sex appeal and beauty. Fear and worry may arise with the lines that emerge, or the sagging of our skin, or the thickening of waistlines or age spots. Maybe we have connected self-esteem to being what we have been told is sexually desirable, or being a fully participating member of society. Our attitudes towards the transition into Second Spring can create distress and pain in our bodies, since what we think and feel exert an energetic influence on both our psyche and soma. Prior to the manifestation of any significant physiological or physical change, an energetic shift will take place. The shift may result from experiencing excessive or inappropriately expressed worry, sadness, fear or anger around the aging process. Over a prolonged period of time, we may have no outlet to express our emotions. We may experience a sense of helplessness or isolation in our capacity to affect change in what we're feeling. We may feel immobilized from fear to even familiarize ourselves with our emotions, or cannot sense what it is that distresses us. Continued emotional distress will move us away from the normal and healthy functioning of our body/mind.

CHANGE AND IMPERMANENCE

We grow up and grow old. We are in the constant process of change. We change every moment. We aren't the same person we were a second ago. Cells have divided and died, we have seen something new, realized an insight, thought a new thought, heard an unfamiliar sound or experienced a feeling. We do not have the same mental content, cellular substance or energy that we had a moment ago. Each moment comes and then goes, and then the next one arises.

We are not the same as we were when we were young women. Nor as young women were we the same as when we were children, and nor will we be the same as we grow into old women. Our lives are a process of continually becoming. It is this process of change that we are so resistant to. The natural movement through life is inevitable and yet so difficult to accept. We want what has passed, or wish for what we don't have. We may reflect on the past happily or with regret and view the future with anticipation or fear. Our lives pass by and we're living in a state of wishing, wanting, fearing or regretting. Our capacity to accept the impermanent nature of existence and live in the present moment will bring us relief from suffering. It is to realize that what we say, do and think in the present moment brings us in touch with our authentic natures.

Impermanence may seem so apparent to us that we tend to forget about it. You may be thinking, of course I know the seasons change and day turns into night. We can accept this. This is so obvious we don't give impermanence any attention. It is more difficult to accept the impermanent nature of our bodies. Perhaps this is because it is not an objective, far-off view of impermanence. It is our subjective experience of imperma- nence on a profoundly intimate level. Our very egos are at stake in this case. We're getting older, with more aches and pains, more wrinkles, less energy. We like to deny our age, and of course the ultimate denial of aging is the denial of death.

If we could see that resisting the impermanence in our lives and in the people and things around us is what brings us our greatest pain, would this be helpful? Can we see how our hold- ing on to our youth, or the health we had at twenty, is causing us great mental distress? Perhaps we may begin to accept the changes that will happen whether or not we flow with them.

LEAH

Leah says getting older is "like sand slipping through her fin- gers." Time is slipping away fast. "I feel like I never have the time for what needs to be done." Leah is fifty-two years old and says she is "getting older and it's the pits." On her fiftieth birthday she cried all day. As flowers and cards arrived, she burst into tears. She thinks of her forties as the best years of her life: she remarried, her daughter graduated from univer- sity and her mother was still alive.

Right now, she sums up her image of the future in this description: "Picture yourself on top of a mountain with skis, and there's no place to go but down." She feels that she is much closer to getting heart disease and diabetes and has to work hard to fight the prospect of aging. She exercises to keep herself in shape and reads to understand what lies ahead. But she can't ignore the loss of memory or her decreased energy or the irritations that surface. She says, "I go blank every once in a while. It's like the computer is overloaded and there's no disk space left." She's finding she doesn't have the capacity to work full-time, do the shopping, clean the house and cook the meals the way she used to.

Leah gets irritated and tells her husband, "Leave me alone when I go into these moods. Don't take it personally." She acknowledges her feelings around the changes that are occurring as she ages and isn't afraid or ashamed to express them; she doesn't want to be seen as a whiner. As she honours her feelings, she is also able to focus on the positive aspects of her life. She is relatively content with work and her family and has a wonderful second husband. She says that if she had one year left to live, she would stop working and make more of an effort to see her friends and relatives more often. She realizes that the people in her life are not going to be around for long, especially her older friends. "I sometimes look at my husband lying on the couch and realize that one day he might not be lying there and I feel more affectionate towards him," she says. "I tell him that I love him. I do this with my daughter and good friends and I make sure to give them a hug. I try to make the time I do have with them better, and in doing this, it is better."

Leah is making the present moment count by connecting with her family and friends. She's been able to transform her resistance to the process of aging into acts of love. The ability to see the impermanence of life brings value to what we hold dear. In Leah's case, acknowledging the transitory quality of life has enabled her to express her love and gratitude to her loved ones. She doesn't wait for a special occasion; she tells them she loves them in that moment. When we embrace the impermanence of all things, we won't be overwhelmed and debilitated. Rather, we can be calm and maintain peace as we face the ups and downs of life.

We look for permanence because we love and desire certainty. If something remains or does not change, then we feel reassured. Unfortunately, we look for certainty in the impermanent nature of existence. It is a losing proposition that brings us great dissatisfaction, suffering and pain. Accepting impermanence isn't really a pessimistic view that says everything will end anyways, so why bother, we're doomed to unhappiness. Like Yin and Yang, there is not only one aspect of impermanence but two. Impermanence offers new possibilities. If we remain static, then we are stuck with whatever we have that we don't want in our lives. And if things didn't change we wouldn't have the potential to achieve what we don't have but want. Impermanence means that our health, or happiness, whatever it is we want, becomes a possibility. There is opportunity for healing and growth.

In Second Spring, accepting the impermanent nature of life will help us heal into the fullness of existence. If we find ourselves resisting our entry into Second Spring, what might we do to help ourselves make this unavoidable transition with ease and compassion? What measures can be taken to empower ourselves?

Our strong emotions are red flags. Like our physical symptoms, they offer us a clue that something significant and dramatic is being experienced. Our insecurity at facing the unknowns that Second Spring may bring to us physically, emotionally and spiritually is often the most difficult part of our journey. The words of the poet T. S. Eliot come to mind:

In order to arrive at what you do not know
  You must go by a way which is the way of ignorance.
In order to possess what you do not possess
  You must go by the way of dispossession.
In order to arrive at what you are not
  You must go through the way in which you are not.
And what you do not know is the only thing you know
And what you own is what you do not own
And where you are is where you are not.

The seeming contradiction in Eliot's poem is the very essence of the concept of Yin and Yang and is a reminder to embrace everything, including the unknown. Wanting to know can make us take action and jump to conclusions. But we should not force something to happen out of fear. In doing this, we perpetuate what we do know and do not allow anything new to develop or emerge.

To me, Eliot's beautiful poem tells us to start where we are. To arrive at a place of acceptance and serenity as we age, the poem suggests we must move through what we are currently experiencing. Sadness or fear may be present, or we may feel relief and excitement. To move through this unknown territory, we don't have to try to eliminate our feelings. When we are in pain or distress, our feelings offer significant information. Our strong emotions carry the seeds of positive energy. The very source of our peaceful older years will be discovered in the difficulties of our transition. The roots of our difficulties are the ground of our compassion, which will be with us for the remainder of our lives.

What are we feeling right now? What we want, perhaps, is the beauty or health or vitality of our younger years. Perhaps it is visibility or independence. We may be angry at our change in status, or our failing memory, or the loss of energy, or our sagging breasts or any of the other myriad changes that may be occurring. Anger is a very significant emotion related to the free movement of energy in a woman. How we deal with our angry feelings is important to the smooth flow of Qi and Blood, and how we support our Liver and Kidneys. Dealing with anger will help make our transition to Second Spring easier and will lead to acceptance and readiness for other changes to come.

I am focusing on anger because I have noticed that in the West anger is very difficult for women to express. Arguably, it is more acceptable for women to show feelings that are culturally regarded as weak, like sadness, fear or disappointment, while men are socialized to use anger to conceal these same emotions. The women I have treated often feel that anger is a negative or "bad" emotion. This viewpoint shows the cultural attitudes that they have internalized. Many women hold in their anger and as a result get depressed. Depression is sometimes referred to as "anger turned inward." People who are depressed often move between being angry at themselves and getting angry with other people.

Since emotions are expressions of Qi, in themselves they are neither good nor bad. In fact, feeling angry for being unjustly treated may be a healing sign of our self-worth and respect. It is our judgment of our feelings, or how we use them, that hinders the free expression of our emotions. We may be afraid to show our anger for fear of being rejected or abandoned. We end up suppressing our feelings as well as our behaviours, and internalizing anger can make us feel powerless, helpless, worthless and unhappy.

In order to deal with our anger, we must first connect with our emotion, that is, know we are feeling angry. One way to do this is to pay attention to what we're feeling in our body. We can focus on our physical state, since it is intimately connected with our emotions. I am not talking about being aware of our body in the way we normally consider it. This is different than reflecting on moisturizing dry patches of skin, or losing five pounds or toning up our muscles. This is feeling and sensing the body as a way to offer insights into our emotional states. Where is my body tensing? Where do I feel contracted in my body? A body scan will help us sense where we may be holding our emotions and will bring us in touch with what we're disconnected from.

BODY SCAN MEDITATION

In scanning the body, we become aware of what we are feeling, make note of it and then let go of the feeling. As we become mindful of the sensations in our body, and the related feelings and thoughts, we are more able to be with whatever we are experiencing in the present moment. Try to do the scan slowly, take at least ten minutes—thirty minutes is a better length of time. Have someone read the following instructions to you slowly, or record yourself reading them and play the tape back as you do the meditation.

———

Sit or lie quietly and begin to connect with how you feel. Close your eyes and breathe deeply. Notice your in-breath and out-breath. Feel where your body is making contact with the bed or the chair or the floor. Keep breathing deeply. Now bring your awareness to your body. Spend time on the different parts, checking to see how each feels. Begin with the toes of your right foot. Can you feel your toes? Notice what sensations are present. Are you experiencing tension, pressure, uneasiness, discomfort or pain, or calm, relaxing sensations? Slowly move your attention up from your toes to your ankle. Flex it if you are having difficulty sensing it. Check to see how it feels. Is your mind thinking, pulling you away from your body? Gently notice where it is and bring your awareness back to your breathing. Slowly bring your awareness up your right leg, up your calf to your knee.

Move your attention to your thigh and up to your hip. Remember to note the subtle sensation or feeling. If there is an uncomfortable feeling, stay with it. Visualize letting go of the uncomfortable feeling. Are there colours you sense with different areas? Witness the sensation you feel, try not to get involved in the "story" attached to the feeling. If you find your attention goes away from your body, simply note that you are thinking about something and bring your awareness back to your body.

At first you may not feel a lot, especially if you are not intimately connected with your feelings. But your body will reveal where your emotions are stored. Do you feel heaviness in your chest or nervousness in your stomach? If you experience uncomfortable feelings or sensations, observe how this feels. Don't try to change the feeling. Try to witness it until it shifts. If you can be with this feeling for long enough, it will move. Allow the feeling, the energy, to move; don't get blocked by your thoughts. The change may be slight, but there will be a change. Stay with the feeling, observe the sensations it brings up in your body. Once you feel the shift, notice the difference in sensation and visualize letting go of the uncomfortableness or pain or tension.

Shift your attention to the toes on your left foot. Slowly move up the ankle, and the calf to the knee. Feel your thigh and move your attention to your hip bone. How do your hips feel now? Are they more relaxed now than when you brought your awareness to them before? Are your hips touching the floor? Are your buttocks touching the chair? How does your lower back feel? If you are feeling uneasy or anxious, bring your awareness to where your body is touching the floor, bed or chair, breathe several breaths and then continue your scan. Keep breathing, deeply inhaling and exhaling.

Shift your attention to your stomach, and move up to your chest and back. Observe any painful sensations, staying with the sensation until it transforms. Take a witness perspective; remove yourself as much as you can from tensing or from the messages you've internalized around the feeling. Trust that the sensation will change. Note the change and visualize letting go of the pain. Can you feel your shoulder blades touching the floor or resting against the back of the chair? Are your shoulders hunched up or are they relaxed? Bring your attention to your neck and up to your head. Scan the features of your head. Are you thinking and going away from your body? Breathe deeply, note that your mind was thinking and return it to your body. Slowly feel your ears, eyes, nose, tongue and mouth. How do your eyes feel? Can you feel the air moving in and out of your nostrils? Are you clenching your teeth? Where is your tongue? Move your attention to the crown of your head. Continue breathing deeply. Now, bring awareness to your entire body. How does it feel? Are you thinking or are you centred on the sensations and feelings in your body? Notice where your mind is. Now, slowly come back to the room. Feel yourself touching the chair, the bed or the floor. Take a deep breath and whenever you feel ready, open your eyes.

This body scan meditation helps us realize that the body and mind are not separate. It helps us describe the sensations and feelings in our physical body and be in touch with our emotions. It will help us develop our ability to connect with the thoughts, beliefs and emotions that drive our experiences. With our awareness, we will know that everything, including our pleasant and unpleasant sensations and feelings, will change.

If we can first get in touch with our anger, then we can make conscious, healthy choices about how we want to express or not express this feeling. Often we have no understanding of how to express our anger assertively. Expression is healthy if we can have our needs filled without hurting others or losing respect for ourselves. Often we lack a model for resolving conflict. If this is the case, we may find ourselves looking for fault in others, making sarcastic comments, indirectly being vindictive, refusing to confront issues, withholding reasons for negative behaviour, or generally being pessimistic.

Consider the story about the young girl who had a very bad temper. Her mother gave her a box of nails and told her to pound a nail into the fence every time she got angry. On the first day, the girl hammered thirty-four nails into the fence. But over time, she drove in fewer and fewer nails. She began to realize that it was easier not to get angry than to pound the nails into the fence. Then, after some time, there was a day when the young girl didn't get angry at all. She went to her mother and reported the good news. Her mother now suggested that for every day she did not lose her temper, she should pull out a nail. After many days had passed, the young girl told her mother with great pride that she had removed all the nails. Her mother took her young daughter's hand and walked to the fence. "My dear, you have worked with your temper very well, but look at this fence, look at the holes. Your angry words can pierce another person and all the 'I'm sorrys' in the world will not matter. The scars will still be there."

We all have wounds from anger—the residue of anger we've vented, and the scars of resentment from the anger inflicted on us. These stay with us for a very long time. As unconscious expressions, they can define who we are. Learning how to express our anger in a way that allows us to grow and is also considerate of ourselves and others allows us to move with our emotions rather than being trapped and victimized by them further. When we feel angry, we can try to sit quietly for ten minutes and notice what is happening in our minds without suppressing our feelings. Don't identify the emotion as "bad" or "good" or reject it. Reflect on what you are feeling and why. Is another person's actions making me angry, or is it something about myself that is making me angry? Since much anger comes from fear, what is it that I am afraid of? Examining our anger to determine where it is coming from can lead us to new perspectives and insights, and helps us connect with our deeply held feelings. Being aware of how we feel helps us make conscious choices, rather than remain stuck in old patterns of behaviour. This moves us forward and helps us make a smooth transition into Second Spring.

FORGIVENESS

In our menopausal years and beyond, many of us strive to become the women we believe we are meant to be. This is a conscious movement towards wholeness. Whatever else we may find, I believe that we will discover respect, love, compassion and forgiveness not just for ourselves but for others as well. I want to focus on forgiveness because by forgiving, we can heal resentment and anger, feelings that are critical to our feminine health. Forgiveness is a spiritual transformation that frees us from resentment. It is an important healer on the levels of Qi and Shen.

Forgiveness is difficult because our egos struggle to be right, or demand justice or retaliation. We sometimes feel that if we forgive someone, we are validating that individual's behaviour. Separating these two concepts is critical. When we forgive, we aren't absolving the other. We are releasing the power that the person or action has over us and taking a step towards being free of our attachment to this particular suffering.

Forgiveness is not something we can force. It seems to

arise when we let go of the past. We surrender the control that our egos exert, and we are no longer controlled by past actions. Forgiveness is not putting forth effort; it involves opening our hearts. It is the realization that we have chosen not to identify with resentment. We are able to see the other beyond the hurt they've caused and thereby move away from it and into a place of greater and deeper healing.

Arguably, forgiveness is more difficult in the West, where we've championed the individual more so than interconnectedness and relationships. The needs of a relationship have to make allowances for what I, as an individual, need. As well, we are generally taught to think in terms of duality: right and wrong, good and bad, you and me, problem and solution. This kind of thinking breeds judgment and comparison. How do we bring this view back into balance? This is the lesson of Yin and Yang, which says we can live in a place of interconnectedness as well as our separate egos. When we think, "We're all in this together," our judgments fall away. We no longer have to hold on to judging others for what they did. We are no different than them. This movement to a new way of seeing an old resentment brings us into the present, as we let go of past hurts and become free of this attachment.

When I think about forgiveness, I think about letting go of resentment, blame and possibly guilt, and accepting the other person even though I may not agree with his or her actions, feelings and thoughts. Sometimes it is very difficult to let go of my beliefs and feelings. I become identified with my point of view, and it feels easier to maintain this position than to soften my grip and open my heart. Forgiveness is not about figuring out whether I'm right, or condemning if the other is wrong. It is realizing what I'm holding on to, and that I no longer want to carry this burden of anger or ill will.

Consider the following parable: There once was a ruler who believed that if he had the answers to three questions, he was sure that he would conduct himself in an appropriate way, regardless of the circumstances. His three questions were:

1. When is the best time to do things?
2. Who are the most important people?
3. What is the most important thing?

He sent out the three questions throughout the land he ruled, requesting his subjects to respond. If he was satisfied with the answers, he would offer the person a generous reward.

None of the responses were satisfactory, so he set out to find the answers himself. He decided to talk to an old master who lived high atop a mountain. When the ruler reached the mountaintop, he asked the master the three questions. The old man was in his garden working. He listened carefully and then resumed digging without uttering a word. The ruler watched the old man and thought, this man looks very tired, so he said, "I'll take over and dig for a while. You take a rest." And so the ruler dug and the master rested. After several hours the ruler put down his shovel and said to the master, "If you do not want to answer my questions, I'll take my leave now."

At that moment the master asked, "Did you hear something?" He looked towards the forest. Suddenly a man came stumbling out of the woods, holding his belly. The master and the ruler ran towards him and saw him fall to the ground. They saw blood on his shirt and ripped it open. There was a deep cut. The ruler cleaned the injury and used his shirt as a bandage. The man opened his eyes and asked if he could have something to drink. The ruler ran to the nearby river and brought some water for the man, who gulped it down and then fell back and slept. The master and the ruler carried the man to the master's hut and gently lay him on the bed. By now, the ruler was also exhausted, so he too fell asleep.

The next morning, when the ruler awoke, the injured man was standing over him, intently gazing down at him. "Forgive me," he said. The ruler sat up, "Forgive you? Forgive you for what?" The man replied, "We have never met, but I have considered you my enemy. In the last war, you killed my brother and confiscated my family's property. I vowed to seek vengeance on behalf of my family. I swore I'd kill you. Yesterday I waited in the woods for you to return down the mountain so that I could finally get revenge. I waited for a long time and still you did not come down, so I came out of the woods to look for you. But instead, your guards saw me and seeing who I was, attacked me, injuring me with this severe wound. I managed to escape, but if you hadn't taken care of me, I would have died. It was my plan to murder you, but instead you saved my life. I feel ashamed and very grateful. Please, will you forgive me?"

The ruler was amazed. "It is good to hear that your hatred has ended. As I hear your story, I too am sorry for the pain I've inflicted on you and your family. War is horrible. I forgive you and I give you back your lands. Let us be friends from now on." The ruler directed his guards to safely return the man to his home. He then said to the master, "I must leave and go back down the mountain. I will continue to search for the answers to my questions. Perhaps one day I will find them. Goodbye."

The master laughed and said, "Your Majesty, your questions have been answered."

"What do you mean?" asked the ruler, surprised.

The master said, "If you had not helped me work in my garden yesterday, you would not have been delayed and you would have been ambushed on your return home. So the most important time for you was the time you spent digging in my garden. And the most important person was me, the person who you were with, and the most important thing for you to do was to simply help me. Later, when the injured man came, the most important time was the time you spent attending to his wound, otherwise he would have died and the opportunity for forgiveness and friendship would have been lost. He was the most important person in that moment and the most important thing to do was to care for his wound. The present moment is the only moment. The most important person is always the person you're with. And the most important thing to do is always to make the person standing beside you happy. What could be simpler or more important?" The ruler bowed in gratitude and left in peace.

This parable teaches us that it is our search for truth and our compassionate responses in the face of suffering that will reveal insights and bring us to forgiveness. How may we open our hearts? How do we let go of the past, come into the present moment and start afresh? This is the challenge we must face and the action we must take.

MEDITATION ON FORGIVENESS

To undertake this practice, which Buddhism offers us, we sit comfortably, closing our eyes. We allow our breath to be natural. We relax our bodies and minds. We breathe deeply several times and bring to mind someone who has hurt us, caused us pain, either knowingly or unknowingly. Inhaling from our hearts, we say, "There are many ways that I have been harmed by others' thoughts, words and actions. There are countless ways that others have hurt and injured me. They have betrayed, caused sadness and abandoned me, consciously and unconsciously, due to their own anger, hurt and confusion. I acknowledge these now. And as much as I am able, I offer forgiveness. As much as I can, I let go of my resentment and anger. I will hold them in my heart." Gently send forgiveness. We do not force ourselves. We may still feel resentful and hurt. So we acknowledge our egos that hold on to our resentment. We accept these feelings and continue to practice this meditation. We remind ourselves this isn't an act of overlooking what others have done to us. It is letting go of our resentment, hurt, sadness and fear, seeing this person in their humanity, in their imperfection. We open our hearts to them and thereby also open our hearts to ourselves.

Now we allow ourselves to remember and visualize how we've hurt others. Breathing in deeply, we repeat, "There are many ways that I have harmed others through my thoughts, words and actions. There are countless ways that I have hurt and injured others. I have betrayed, caused sadness and abandoned them, consciously and unconsciously, due to my own anger, hurt and confusion. I acknowledge these now. I ask forgiveness of others. May I be forgiven." We ask forgiveness, not coloured with guilt, but with the understanding that we are not perfect. We try to let go of self-criticism. We soften our hearts and ask for forgiveness with the intention of letting go all that has come between us and other people.

Finally, we offer forgiveness to ourselves. If we can truly give love to ourselves we will be able to then receive love from another. Can we acknowledge that we have faults, but that we are not just our faults? That we don't always do things perfectly, but we do the best we can? Breathing in deeply, repeat, "There are many ways that I have harmed myself through my thoughts, words and actions. There are countless ways that I have hurt and injured myself. I have betrayed, caused sadness and abandoned myself, consciously and unconsciously, due to my own anger, hurt and confusion. I acknowledge these now. I offer forgiveness to myself. May I be forgiven." Breathe in love and forgiveness into your heart and feel the healing power of giving this to yourself.

Sometimes we feel that forgiveness is beyond our capacity. We cannot forgive. However, this transformational process is, in fact, vital to our spiritual healing. If we let go of our egos, we are able to become whole and vital in all areas of our being. The other person does not have to accept our forgiveness, nor does anyone have to forgive us for what we've done. Forgiveness requires only our involvement. It frees our hearts and stops the cycle of hurt and resentment. It opens us up into connection and relationship. It is an act of compassionate acceptance of ourselves and others.

EXPERIENCING ACCEPTANCE

My journey to accepting myself is fundamentally rooted in

my relationship with my grandmother. She looked after me from the time I was two until the age of six because the Communist government sent my father to work in another city, and my mother to a re-education farm. When I was three, my grandmother enrolled me in kindergarten. I remember her taking me to school that first day, before she went to work. When I realized she was going to leave me, I started to cry and begged her not to go. In my desperation to hold on to her, I bit her hand and held on with all the strength I could muster. The teachers were yelling, but I would not let go. I tore the flesh on her hand and drew blood. I began to sob hysterically. My grandmother kept telling the teachers, "Don't scare her, she wants to be with me. It's OK." Before she left, she said, "Don't hurt her, I'll be back."

The bite I'd given her was so bad she had to go to the hospital for twelve stiches! When she returned to the kindergarten to pick me up, she smiled and said that when she'd reported to work, she was told she could go home because of her wound. "I don't have to go to work for three days, so we can stay at home together!" she announced.

My grandmother understood my three-year-old terror and accepted me unconditionally. It seemed that whatever I did, she responded with care and concern for my welfare. I remember another occasion when I was very naughty. In the late 1950s, a person in Kunming would be very lucky to own one knitted sweater. My grandmother had one handmade sweater in her wardrobe. One day, I picked up a pair of scissors and proceeded to cut right up the back of it, through each of the hand-knit stitches! When my brother and sisters saw what I'd done, they began chastising me, but my grandmother quickly

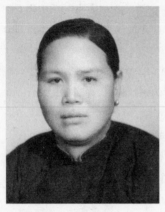

My grandmother

came to my defence. She said, "Yelling at her will have no effect. It is only a sweater. Just talk to her and tell her that this is not proper behaviour and she is not to do it again." She said to me, "In fact, I think you are able to use scissors very well." I started to cry and said I was sorry.

My grandmother had the wisdom to separate my behaviour from who I was, and didn't try to make me feel that I was a bad child for some of the naughty things I did. She took the opportunity to teach me rather than punish me, and I am eternally grateful for her unconditional love and acceptance. I feel that her nurturing of me instilled the confidence and self-esteem that I have drawn upon throughout my life.

Carl Rogers, the founder of humanistic psychology, coined the phrase "unconditional positive regard," and said it was fundamental to the process of becoming fulfilled. When he talked about unconditional positive regard, he was referring to caring and nonjudgmental acceptance unburdened with sentimentality, possessiveness or an agenda. When we are able to experience unconditional positive regard, we feel we are being accepted for who we are. We are cared for without being evaluated or judged for what we feel or do. This allows us to be separate and independent people. We develop unconditional positive regard (self-esteem) for ourselves, and can accept ourselves.

Being who we are involves accepting all of what we embody. Self-acceptance allows us to acknowledge all of our thoughts, words, actions and feelings without denial, repudiation or avoidance. We open to embracing all aspects of our being, the parts we like and the parts we don't. We accept our imperfections and humanity without conditions.

So often we try to ignore, deny or suppress the fullness of our humanity, by wanting only happiness, success, health and youth in our lives. When we become aware of our non-acceptance, we gain insight into the nature of existence. We are not perfect. Nothing is perfect. Existence is not perfect. Life is not always fair, nor satisfactory, nor kind. Nor is it always unfair, unsatisfactory or unkind. Existence changes. It is not absolute. We cannot say that life is always secure and safe, but we can watch our tendency to want it to be. We can watch how we structure our inner and outer worlds to assure ourselves that we are secure and safe. We can observe our desire to accept only one perspective over another. And we know that if we embrace the fullness of all, Yin and Yang, we will move towards wholeness. Shifting to this wide-angle view, a unitary perspective, allows us to accept the transitory nature of existence.

Thus, our relationship with Second Spring can keep us in harmonious relationships with ourselves and with others, as well as within a larger context. As we open to our spirituality, to forgiveness, to acceptance of ourselves, we open to new possibilities, to the time of our Second Spring—a time when our creativity is renewed and new growth begins, is nurtured and embraced.

CHAPTER SEVENTEEN

A Natural Transition

For me, the word *menopause*, and not the natural life transition it is referring to, conjures up an impending disease, a series of afflictions that require medical intervention. This is a misconception and popular belief that I know I have absorbed from Western society. What is known in the West as menopause is, in China, basically a non-event. It is seen as a harbinger of old age, a greatly respected life stage and a natural progression in life's journey.

My mother was fifty years old when the flow of her Heavenly Water became irregular. For the next five years, her period would arrive for a few cycles and then stop for a few months. By the age of fifty-five, her menses ceased completely. As a typical Chinese woman, she did not expect, nor did she experience, hot flashes, night sweats, insomnia, depression or fatigue during this time. The only significant symptom that accompanied her transition was irritability. She noticed that on occasion she was more bad-tempered with my father and us children than she had been before.

In moving to the nonreproductive stage of her life, my mother did not undertake any changes in her diet or lifestyle, nor did she purposefully set out to maintain the status quo in her life. She did not regard the passage into Second Spring as a time of upheaval or as a stage requiring special consideration. In fact, she looked forward to her nonreproductive years as a time of rejuvenation, of new possibilities and potential.

The natural transition into Second Spring does not automatically bring painful and afflicting symptoms, but possibly gradual and progressive ones. This is not to discount that changes will occur, but, like my mother, there are some of us who will experience little, perhaps no, discomfort. Because in the West we've been conditioned to associate menopause with illness and a need for medical intervention or supplementation, we may feel apprehensive and afraid of the natural changes that occur. Perhaps the medicalization of menopause is partly the result of women seeking treatment for the relief of symptoms. Consequently, menopause is often perceived as the cause of debilitating difficulties for women in mid-life. Many of us expect and wait for things to go wrong. And what we anticipate is often what we experience. If we expect negative symptoms, then we will look for them. We may end up using menopause as a catch-all for many discomforts and difficulties that are not even related to this transition.

BERNIE

When Bernie first came to my office, she was a fifty-one-year-old schoolteacher transitioning into her Second Spring. She found she couldn't sleep and her insomnia had led to a loss of appetite. Everything tasted like wood chips to her. She said, "I feel like someone is standing on my sternum with a huge stone underfoot, pressing into my chest. There's tremendous tension in my eyes and they feel like they're being pulled inwards, inside my head. One day I was lying on my couch, and I could feel my body tremble and shake at every slightest sound. I didn't feel like I could speak and whatever I did say didn't sound believable."

Bernie was in a severe state of depression, which her family doctor associated with menopause. But there were many stressful factors converging on her at this point in her life. She had fallen in love with a man, who though unmarried, was not in love with her. He could not forget his first wife, who had passed away, and open himself up to Bernie. At the same time, her youngest daughter was leaving home. And at school, she was having difficulties with a problematic student who was disobedient and abusive and continually disrupting classes. Bernie felt worthless; she felt that she had not achieved anything of value in her life and that all her efforts had been a waste. She engaged in harsh self-criticism. Her inner voice kept saying, "How could you do this, Bernie? You are fully engaged in your life, so how can you feel like this?"

It was through practising yoga and "just getting tired of being miserable" that helped Bernie move through her depression. But she went on to experience two subsequent bouts over the next two decades. Though triggered by a series of different circumstances, the experiences were the same. She was debilitated and unable to sleep and function. Deciding whether to clean her glasses became a stressful undertaking and simple things became overwhelming.

Bernie started to see a counsellor and came to realize that her self-loathing was rooted in the physical abuse she'd received as a child at the hands of her mother. From the time she was five or six, her mother beat her with a razor strap, leaving welts. Eventually, Bernie began to internalize her mother's judgment of her. She remembers getting grass stains on her white socks and repeating, "Bad Bernie, bad Bernie."

Through the help of her counsellor and her family, Bernie started to work through her childhood issues. She realized that though her depression and entry into Second Spring had occurred simultaneously, her illness was not part of her menopausal symptoms.

At mid-life, when we typically transition into Second Spring, there are often a number of stresses contributing to our emotional and physical loads, such as tending to the needs of our declining parents, adjusting to changed roles in the home or workplace, dealing with children leaving home, retiring from our professions, experiencing mental and physical changes in body image and so on. If we have internalized negative stereotypes of menopausal women, then we can easily attribute the distress and discomfort of other stress factors in our lives to menopause.

However, many of us *will* experience some very real physical symptoms during our transition into Second Spring. As Spleen function declines there is less Blood, Qi and other body fluids available to hydrate the body. We experience this reduction in moisture as vaginal dryness and discomfort, as well as dry hair, skin, eyes and nails. Also we may become constipated. As our Yin declines and is no longer able to balance out our Yang, the excess Yang takes the form of Heat, which rises or vents upwards and towards the head and shoulders and the surface of the body, resulting in hot flashes and night sweats. These symptoms may also affect our capacity for sound sleep. Some of us will wake up sweating during our sleeping hours and need to rise to change our clothing. Without sufficient rest, we may become easily irritated and bad-tempered, and experience a loss of energy. This condition may be exacerbated if we have a blockage of Qi in our Liver system, which will aggravate a Blood Deficiency. Obstructed Liver Qi has a tendency to transform into Heat, and if Heat moves in fits and starts, we may express anger or irritation in bursts that may be inappropriate to the circumstances. Anger is a hot emotion, as is reflected when we speak of "burning with rage," or "making my blood boil" or "blowing off steam" or "her fiery temper."

Weakened Blood may also affect the supply of Blood to the Heart. If the Heart does not receive sufficient Blood and Yin, it cannot ground the Shen, the most refined energy that is associated with the mind or Spirit. If Shen is not rooted, we may find difficulty in remembering or formulating our thoughts. We may also become easily agitated, feel anxious and have difficulty sleeping or enjoying restful sleep.

The slowing down of the Spleen's functioning is another contributing factor to the weight gain that many of us complain of at this stage of our lives. A weakened Spleen will manifest as weight accumulation particularly around the middle torso, the hips and waist. Often, those of us with Spleen Qi Deficiencies will feel tired after we eat, and may have a tendency to worry excessively. Western medical science generally views weight gain as directly tied to overeating and recommends eating less. In Chinese medicine, weight is not managed by dieting. Although Chinese medicine practitioners consider the types and quantities of foods eaten, the focus is on the imbalances in the relevant Organ systems.

Over time, the decline in Kidney Yin will affect the functioning of the Kidney Organ system and may give rise to a weakening of Kidney Yang energy as well. It is primarily Kidney Yin and Yang Deficiencies that contribute to the symptoms of aging. The Kidneys govern the Marrow, ears, the Bladder and hair. As we get older, these areas decline in functioning due to the weakening of our Kidney energy. Marrow in TCM refers to the bone marrow, brain, spinal cord and bones. Since Essence is needed for the production of Marrow, weakened Kidneys will not be able to sufficiently nourish the brain, leading to a loss of memory, poor concentration, reduced ability to think and impaired vision. Healthy Marrow also underlies the formation of bone marrow that produces strong bones and teeth. This is the reason that as we age, we often experience loss of bone density, arthritis and dental problems. Kidney weakness also manifests as impaired hearing, including tinnitus, ringing in the ears and problems controlling our Bladder. The rich colour, thickness and quality of our hair reflects the strength of our Kidney Essence. These changes, a direct result of Kidney Yin and/or Yang Deficiency and the diminishment of Essence, progress gradually. They reflect the normal process of aging.

The severity of our symptoms will be determined by how well we have nurtured and nourished our Kidneys, conserved our Essence and taken care of our feminine health overall. Our constitutional makeup, or the quality of our parents' Essence when we were conceived, along with our emotional health, diet and lifestyle choices up to this point in our lives are all influential factors in our Kidney health. The Kidneys are associated with the emotion fear, and if we have experienced extended periods of fear and anxiety, or hold this as an underlying state of being, our Kidneys will be weakened. But if we have been careful, in our pre–Second Spring years, to deal with emotional stress, get adequate rest, eat a proper diet and avoid overwork, inordinate physical exertion, frequent childbirths and chronic illnesses, and if we have built up our postnatal Essence to an abundant level, our prenatal Essence will be well-preserved and strong, and our transition to Second Spring will be relatively easy and not problematic.

ANITA

Anita was fifty-four when her periods stopped abruptly. She did not undergo a lengthy transition. The only irregularity in her flow of Heavenly Water before its cessation was a heavy period two cycles prior to ending. She did not experience hot flashes or night sweats. The only changes she noticed were a slight loss in her ability to remember and her sleep was not as deep. Basically, however, her transition was a non-event that did not bring her any degree of discomfort.

Anita's diet consisted of tofu, chicken and fresh fruit and vegetables, and her habit was to eat small meals every two hours. She did not eat dairy products or red meat. In addition, she took nutritional supplements, such as evening primrose oil, vitamins E and C, along with a multivitamin, CoQ10, a

B-complex vitamin, calcium and magnesium with Vitamin D3, and gingko. For exercise, she ran daily, did yoga and lifted weights.

Anita considers her husband her best friend and they continue to enjoy a satisfying sex life. Her attitude is to let go of problems that she has no control over. She also tries not to hold on to issues that she has already voiced concerns about. She feels that life has been good to her and focuses on the positive aspects. When she was in her twenties and thirties, Anita cared what others thought of her and tried to please her family and friends. As she has aged, she feels she has gained more confidence, maturity and experience. This has helped her to accept herself and care less about the opinions of others. In transitioning to Second Spring, Anita's healthy emotional life and her self-care supported and contributed to a relatively symptom-free transition.

You may be thinking, "According to TCM, I haven't taken care of my body, heart and mind so far in my life." Or perhaps you feel that you were not endowed with a strong constitution. You may already be having problems with this life transition and feel that your past choices were not the best. Don't worry; it is not too late to affect changes to your health and well-being. Even though the focus of Chinese medicine is on prevention, there is still much we can do to improve our emotional, physical and spiritual lives in our Second Spring. Appropriate measures and specific lifestyle changes need not be major, but they can greatly ease us through this transition.

HELPING OURSELVES

The gradual and integrated approach of Chinese medicine can be extremely beneficial as we move from our reproductive to our nonreproductive years. Though TCM recommendations are not necessarily quick fixes, they are natural, gentle and safe and can be effective in eliminating or reducing symptoms that may arise from the imbalances in our bodies as our Organ systems naturally begin to weaken with age and we experience the cumulative effect of the choices we have made in our lives.

Symptoms related to menopause may be eliminated or reduced by avoiding lifestyle choices that decrease the functioning of the Kidneys, and by undertaking any measures that support this Organ system and facilitate the free movement of Qi. Typical of Chinese medicine, recommendations prevent unnecessary erosion or consumption of our Essence. The practices also work to build postnatal Essence and bring Yin and Yang back into balance. These recommendations may sound like common sense, and in fact, they are. However, my experience has been that "common sense" is not always common. Given the demands of modern life, common sense practices are often difficult to carry out. For example, one of the most important considerations during menopause is to try not to get too stressed, overtired or overworked—not such an easy accomplishment.

DIET

Diet is one way that we can proactively support our Kidney system and other Organ networks. We should eat nutritiously balanced meals at regular intervals. The quantity of food we consume is also important. Overeating can tax our Spleen, and undereating or dieting can reduce the amount of Blood and Qi that is produced. Try not to eat after 8 P.M., since any food that you eat late at night may remain in your Stomach as you sleep. This will further burden the Spleen and give rise to digestive problems and inefficient absorption and contribute to weight gain.

In addition, if we consume Cold or raw foods and drinks, the Spleen will have to work harder or draw upon the Kidneys for additional Qi, or Heat, to transform and transport the food. The body will also have to produce more Heat to counterbalance the Cold, leading to less moisture and increased hot flashes.

Since Qi flows through the Stomach and Spleen systems between 7 and 11 A.M., it is particularly important to eat a breakfast that is agreeable to these Organs, such as warm

TABLE 6: DIETARY RECOMMENDATIONS FOR SECOND SPRING

AVOID OR MINIMIZE EATING	EAT
• Cold foods and drinks • Frozen foods • Raw foods • Dairy products • Rich, fatty foods • Greasy foods • Sugar and refined carbohydrates • Coffee • Alcohol • Carbonated soft drinks • Hot and spicy foods • Large amounts of red meat	• Cooked foods that are served warm • Lightly cooked, fresh vegetables • Dark green leafy vegetables, dried longan fruit, liver, eggs, raisins • Almonds, walnuts, sunflower seeds, pumpkin seeds • Bone soups • Soy products • String beans, kidney beans, black beans • Mung beans and sprouts • Black sesame seeds • Seaweed • Oily fish such as sardines, salmon, tuna, mackerel • Whole grains

cooked foods. It is recommended that we avoid eating rich, fatty foods or greasy foods and minimize the amount of dairy products we ingest. Table 6 on the preceding page summarizes TCM dietary recommendations for Second Spring.

EXERCISE

Regular exercise is beneficial in circulating Qi and Blood. In China, physical activity is regarded as an indispensable component and expression of health. Without movement on a daily basis, our Qi will not flow smoothly, and we will become out of balance, physically as well as emotionally. If our emotions are blocked, our Qi may stagnate. Those of us with an inclination to anger, frustration or irritability would be wise to exercise regularly to keep our Qi moving.

Exercise also stimulates the Spleen and benefits the Lungs. It can help us deal with the symptoms of menopause and the natural aging process. Exercising can improve our aches and pains. If we choose to exercise out of doors, we may find that the fresh air is invigorating and helps us sleep better. The weight that we naturally gain at this time may seem more manageable, and we may become more regular in our bowel movements. It is also a way to work with depression, as it can improve our overall sense of well-being.

Because high-impact exercises, such as aerobics and jogging, can exhaust Qi and contribute to a further deficiency of Blood and Yin, we may want to rethink the type of exercise we engage in. Walking, cycling, swimming, dancing and stretching are all good ways of keeping active. Our regular daily activities, such as cleaning the house, working in the garden and washing the car, are also good forms of exercise.

Yoga, Tai Chi and Qi Gong are particularly helpful in conserving Essence and building energy while providing aerobic enhancement through breathing and weight-bearing exercise. Their benefits are similar to those of high-impact exercises, but without the stress and strain on the body. These practices are focused on balancing us physically, mentally and spiritually, which is beneficial as we transition and experience energetic disharmonies and symptoms.

TAI CHI

Tai Chi is a particularly beneficial form of exercise. From the age of thirty, my mother had painful arthritis in her knee. She believes that the condition developed from working on the re-education farm for many years and living in damp conditions. In her early thirties, the pain was so severe that there were times when she needed help to walk. By the time she was thirty-five, my mother had started to practise Tai Chi. Within two to three years, her knee was significantly better. She was able to walk on her own and the pain had subsided.

Throughout the next four decades, my mother continued her practice. She says that Tai Chi not only helped her arthritis but alleviated pain in her neck and ailments in her stomach. Today she spends one hour practising Tai Chi exercises in the park each day. She has taught many people who approach her there with a desire to learn this ancient art. She devotes another hour a day to stretching exercises and walks around the park near her home. My mother maintains that she is walking faster and stronger today than she was forty years ago.

Tai Chi involves cultivating Qi, which tends to become deficient as we age. It uses breathing to improve energy levels, and

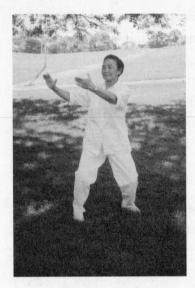

My mother practising Tai Chi
in Toronto

physical movements to circulate energy and help remove blockages. Rather than using muscle energy, it uses our life force, Qi. Through continued practice, our Qi actually increases.

Grounded in Taoism, with its central principle of transformation and change, the movements of Tai Chi are slowed down and flow like water, so that an ending point transforms into the beginning of the next movement, and the completion of this posture gives rise to another step. As well, once a movement reaches its extreme, as when all our weight is on one leg, it shifts to the reverse, and our weight is transferred to the other leg. This is the fullness of Yang changing to Yin and vice versa. I find Tai Chi movement a wonderful metaphor for transitioning to Second Spring. This stage of our feminine cycle is a reflection of the maturity that comes at this point in our lives. We are able to see that what we do has consequences in other aspects of our lives. The way we cared for ourselves during Heavenly Water, through our pregnancies, and during Golden Month will bear fruit during this time, in much the same way that one movement leads to the next in Tai Chi.

At first it feels that we are moving away from Yang, the active energy of youth, to Yin, the receptive energy of old age. But as the name Second Spring implies, this is a time of rebirth, reflowering and further growth. And so the energy shifts back again to Yang. As we grow older, we look inside to find out what it is we want and seek the answers to our questions. Everything is within us. It is like working with Tai Chi.

Tai Chi has the capacity to strengthen connective tissues and so improve our range of movement and relieve pain. And it does not require any specialized equipment or clothing and can be practised anywhere. One need not be young, or fit, or healthy or rich to practise Tai Chi.

Another important advantage is that Tai Chi develops the mind. Because the focus is internal, unlike regular aerobic and muscular exercise, Tai Chi helps to enhance concentration, improve self-perception, bring greater self-awareness and increase positive thinking. The self-confidence and alleviation of tension that results from experiencing these benefits is a significant factor in our overall sense of well-being. In this way, Tai Chi is a moving meditation that enhances the Three Treasures—Essence, Qi and Shen. It is an exceptionally supportive self-care practice that we may undertake as we transition into our Second Spring.

ACUPRESSURE

Acupressure massage can be used to stimulate the flow of Qi and Blood and unblock obstructions. By pressing specific points, we can lead Qi to areas of Deficiency and drain it from areas of Excess, regulating its flow through the Meridians. Either we or someone else can apply steady pressure to the points Yong Quan (see page 96), San Yin Jiao (see page 97) and Zu San Li (see page 98) for up to two minutes once a day. If there is tension or resistance, try pushing a little harder. If the point feels tender, it is probably blocked. This should pass as you continue this practice.

SELF-MASSAGE

Self-massage is another effective way to help move Qi and Blood through the internal Organs. The following massages will assist in providing an adequate supply of Qi and Blood to the Spleen, which weakens with the natural aging process. They are also beneficial in preventing the Bowels from stagnating. If possible, do these massages for five to ten minutes daily.

1. Lie on your back with your legs straight. Starting at the centre of your body, press your fingers under the bottom of your right ribs. Continue doing this, following the bottom edge of your ribs, till you reach below your floating ribs (see illustrations below). Repeat this three times. Do the same series of moves on the left side.

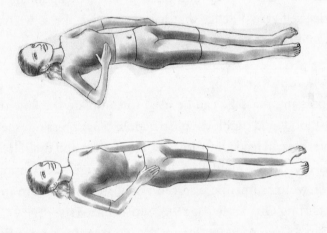

2. Start above your pubic bone and press down with
   your hands. Move your hands upwards towards the ribs
   on your right side, pressing and holding for a count of
   six (see illustrations below). This will track the path of
   the ascending colon. Repeat this three times.

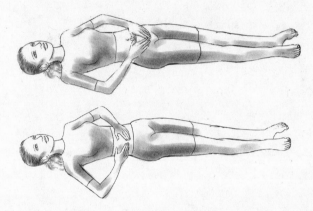

3. Start below the sternum and press down the centre
   of the torso to above the pubic bone (see illustrations
   below). Repeat this three times.

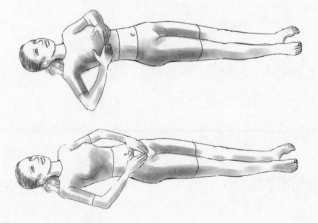

4. Starting on the right side of the belly, press across in a straight line over the abdomen from right to left (see illustrations below). Repeat three times.

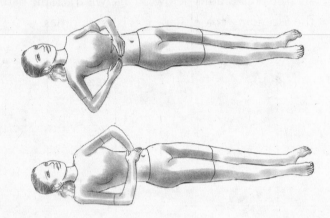

5. Starting from a point on the left side at the waist, press down the side of the abdomen, finishing above the pubic bone (see illustrations below). This follows the course of the descending colon. Do this three times.

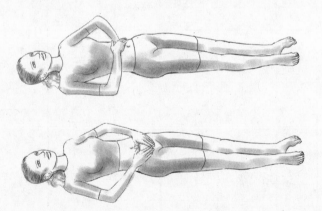

If there are any areas that are tender or sore, go back and massage them once again. Over time, the pain will disappear. Releasing energetic obstructions is very beneficial in preventing further dysfunction that may arise from imbalances.

PUBOCOCCYGEAL EXERCISES

During Second Spring, we may experience a reduction or loss of bladder control, since the Kidneys govern the Bladder. Exercising the pubococcygeal muscle will improve the muscle tone of the pelvic floor and prevent or reduce problems with incontinence. It will also improve our sexual functioning and pleasure. Please check that you are using the correct muscle either by paying attention to the muscle you use to stop your urine flow in midstream, or by placing a finger in your vagina and tightening the muscles around it.

This exercise can be done lying, sitting or standing. Tighten the muscle that you previously identified for five to ten seconds. Slowly release. Repeat ten times. If you are experiencing incontinence from weakened muscles, do several sets of this exercise throughout the day.

ADDITIONAL SELF-CARE PRACTICES

Additional self-care practices to undertake during Second Spring are to go to sleep at the same time each evening and have a sound, undisturbed sleep. Take care not to overwork or overtax yourself physically, mentally and emotionally. If possible, avoid tobacco products and second-hand smoke, as they tend to dry up body fluids and Yin. Also, minimize the use of drugs such as cortisone, diuretics and antacids.

———

These self-care recommendations will help bring balance to our bodies. Remember that there is no need to strive for perfection in undertaking them. Developing regimes comprising healthy recommendations is of limited use if we become stressed. There is a potential for us to get too much of a good thing if our practice creates disharmony.

Some of us may feel that we cannot maintain a regular practice, and so there's no point in doing them at all. In this case, perhaps we can develop an intention towards our good health and well-being. Say to yourself, "It is my intention to be healthy and free of stress, to move through this natural transition with ease. I intend to support myself by taking care of my body, heart and mind." By focusing on our intention, I believe we increase the possibility that we will seriously consider some of these recommendations and integrate them into our daily lives.

HORMONE REPLACEMENT THERAPY RECONSIDERED

In July 2002, the National Institutes of Health (NIH) announced the discontinuation of their study into the effects of Hormone Replacement Therapy (HRT) (using estrogen and progestin) due to increased risks to the study participants with no counterbalancing benefits. Compared to placebo users, the hormone supplement users had higher incidences of strokes, heart attacks, blood clots and an increased risk of breast cancer. Understandably, after the results of this study were announced, my clinic received a higher than normal volume of calls and visits from women uncertain and confused about whether they should continue to take their hormone supplements.

Remembering that we are each unique and have our own special needs, we must make our own decisions. It is important to evaluate our personal risk and benefit factors. Do we have a family history of breast cancer, uterine cancer, uterine fibroids, breast cysts, Alzheimer's, heart attacks, strokes, high cholesterol or high blood pressure? Taking HRT could increase your risk for these conditions. Not taking HRT could increase your risk for osteoporosis and extreme menopausal symptoms such as hot flashes, night sweats, vaginal dryness, mood swings, increased weight and low libido.

HRT offers faster relief from these symptoms than Chinese medicine does. However, HRT does not address the root cause of the symptoms, nor does it strengthen the Kidneys. Theoretically, ancient Chinese medicine practitioners would not condone its use since it makes our bodies think we are still ovulating. It activates the endometrium, resulting in withdrawal bleeding on a regular cycle. The cessation of our menstrual cycle is our bodies' natural means of preventing a further loss of Essence. With prolonged bleeding, our Kidneys, Spleen and Liver are taxed and ultimately depleted, contrary to the natural events that should be occurring in our bodies.

The impact of long-term use of HRT is a Deficiency in Blood (specifically related to the Heart and Liver), Spleen Qi and possibly overall Qi; as well, it can cause Kidney disorders. These imbalances may manifest as hearing or sight problems, insomnia, uterine prolapse and the possibility of diseases associated with our older years, such as Alzheimer's or Parkinson's. The Stagnation of Qi can also result in Blood Stagnation and an increased incidence of Blood clot formation. Since the Liver governs and controls Qi, it can become overtaxed in overseeing the unnatural cycle of bleeding. Obstructions in the flow of Liver Qi can give rise to breast diseases. Moreover, Stagnation of Liver Qi may result in Stagnation of Blood in the pelvic area. This may result in uterine diseases. Often, Stagnation of Qi in the chest area, with symptoms such as angina, can be attributed to Stagnation of energy in the Liver system.

The TCM approach for addressing menopausal symptoms are the dietary recommendations and lifestyle changes given on pages 284 to 294, as well as acupuncture treatments and herbal formulations that nourish the Kidneys, harmonize Yin and Yang and target an individual's specific Organ imbalances. I have worked with many women who have used both Chinese treatments and recommendations and HRT. In treating patients, I acknowledge how debilitating some symptoms can be and, in these instances, understand the patients' desire to use HRT. However, I would advise that taking it be a short-term solution only. After a few months of TCM, many patients wean themselves off HRT by gradually reducing their dosage over a period of time. Stopping HRT abruptly may result in rebound bleeding, hot flashes or other health problems due to the body's dependence on this unnatural form of supplementation.

It is important to raise a few other considerations for those women using HRT. Our experience and results of hormone replacement will be different depending on our dose and method of administration (oral pills, transdermal patches, vaginal hormone creams, intramuscular injections or subcutaneous pellets). Generally, HRT adopts a one-size-fits-all approach, and individual needs aren't considered. Most often we are not prescribed the lowest dosage that is effective for us.

But the biggest factor in how we experience HRT is whether the hormones are synthetic or natural. Synthetic hormones generally have a structure that is similar, but not identical, to the hormones our bodies produce. Therefore they work differently in our bodies and have been found to result in unfavourable effects with possible health risks.

Natural hormones are identical in chemical structure to the hormones produced by our bodies. They come from the urine of pregnant mares—hardly a natural substance for human bodies. Therapy using natural hormones, however, does not evidence the same possibility for adverse effects as synthetic hormone replacement, since the body does not perceive them as foreign substances. Natural hormones are not readily purchased over the counter—pharmaceutical companies cannot patent natural substances, and so doctors are primarily familiar with the drugs marketed to them by large companies, and not the natural alternatives.

Whatever form of treatment you choose, keep in mind that you can always switch if problems arise. As well, please remember that the transition into Second Spring is a natural progression that doesn't require a full-scale offensive against our bodies. If we take care of the different levels of our being, we can increase the possibility of an optimal experience of menopause with minimal unnatural interference or complications.

OUR SEXUAL LIVES

Since, in the West, sex and physical attractiveness are believed to be the property of the young, there is a belief that the sex lives of post-menopausal women are non-existent. We have no desire for sex, and are no longer sexually attractive. These negative perceptions may inhibit our ability to function as whole individuals and satisfy our natural needs. We may actually feel societal pressure to lose interest in sex. When we feel sexual desire, we may become anxious. If we are experiencing sexual problems, we may feel reluctant to discuss them. Or maybe we use these misconceptions as a good excuse not to have a sex life after a long period of disinterest. Is a lack of interest the result of infrequent sexual activity or the cause of it?

The truth is that women's interest in sex continues long after menopause. In fact, many women experience greater sexual desire during the time of Second Spring. Why? The concern of pregnancy has been lifted. With children gone from the family home, there is increased freedom and spontaneity. Women often experience a surge in self-confidence as they "come into their own power," unconstrained by the expectations of others.

Remaining sexually active involves consideration of physical changes, emotional well-being and life circumstances. We may experience discomfort during intercourse due to decreased vaginal moisture or when the lining of the vagina thins. It is important to note that this does not change our capacity to orgasm. The sexual organs, including the clitoris, remain sensitive. One of the most beneficial ways to ease discomfort and pain is to engage in frequent sexual intercourse rather than refrain from it. This helps stimulate our body's natural lubrication. We can also use personal lubricants that are readily available in pharmacies to ease personal discomfort.

Sometimes we may feel rejected and angry in response to a natural decline in sexual activity by our partners. If we are unable to be candid with each other, there is an increased

possibility of doubt about sexual adequacy. We may find ourselves suppressing desire because of the anger and hurt or
rejection that we experience. Honest, open, nonjudgmental
communication will facilitate understanding of the doubts
that arise about performance. We may find that our partner
cannot meet some of our desires, but talking will help us to
make allowances.

Our ability to express what pleasures and satisfies us is
equally critical to hearing what pleasures and satisfies our
partner. Through open communication we can discover ways
to adjust to changes, such as taking more time for foreplay or
expanding the scope of love-making beyond coitus. Building
an intimate relationship is a strong foundation from which to
work through sexual concerns that may arise, and assist in the
transitioning process relative to life changes.

A primary challenge for women as we age is the lack of
available partners. There is a greater possibility that post-
menopausal women will be widowed compared to men of a
similar age. As well, older single women have less of a tendency to remarry relative to older single men. There may also
be greater cultural acceptance of men having relationships
with younger women versus women romantically involved
with younger men. Even though we have experienced more
freedom of sexual expression over the past three to four
decades, we are still living with the perceptions and misconceptions that older women are disinterested in sex. These cultural
stereotypes regarding post-menopausal women and sexual
behaviour can exert a powerful influence on our thinking,
actions, reactions and experiences. Getting in touch with our
sexuality and developing ways to deal with the misconceptions

will help us shift away from the perception that we are non-sexual beings. We can understand how or if we believe in the negative attitudes and become educated about the normal physical changes that occur as we age. Sexual problems are not necessarily a natural aspect of getting older. Sexual activity is a healthy and normal expression of being an adult human. We are capable of being sexual individuals and enjoying the shared intimacy and affection of sex throughout our lives.

SUMMARY

The transition into Second Spring involves a natural progression of changes. The cessation of our Heavenly Water is a result of our bodies' inherent intelligence to preserve our Essence. As our Jing naturally declines, the innate wisdom of our bodies redirects Essence so we are no longer focused on reproduction and instead have more energy and Blood to support our Heart and spiritual journey. As we naturally move from Yin energy into Yang, we venture from our mothering and nurturing roles in search of our place in the world, and what it is we want and need. As well, it is a time for supporting our Yin nature as we seek to fulfill our deeper spiritual needs, potential and aspirations.

The transition to Second Spring can be a confusing, liberating or difficult phase of our lives. Our experience will be determined by numerous factors. Some are within our sphere of influence, others are not. Understanding what we are able to affect is an important step towards feeling empowered and preventing dysfunction and distress. Also, those of us who dread aging may gain a new perspective on our menopausal years. We may begin to see them as a doorway into new possibilities.

Awareness of what we can do to support ourselves can greatly ease our transition. As our Organ systems naturally decline, there are many self-care practices that can help optimize their functioning and strength. Carefully balance your striving to do it all with feeling as though it requires too much effort—otherwise it becomes yet another problem.

TCM is about bringing harmony into our lives. Viewing ourselves through this filter is in itself a huge self-care practice.

Recognizing how hard we push ourselves or how much we relinquish is a wonderful first step towards reclaiming harmony and a new state of balance. By doing this we begin to focus on our experiences and expressions of health. Even though the recommendations make sense, why don't I want to follow them? What is stopping me? We start to move from focusing on the symptoms towards a search for the energetic source of our reluctance, our drive, our distress. We are practising Chinese medicine—we are using our symptoms to gain further information about ourselves, to ease ourselves back into balance.

I feel this is a significant step as it shifts our relationship with our symptoms. Our pain, our discomfort, our strong feelings are not the enemy to be eradicated. They are as much a part of us as our health, happiness and vitality. As we explore our feelings around our symptoms or our loss of interest in sex, our anger at being invisible or our sagging breasts, we open to a greater acceptance of all aspects of who we are. We move into the realm of our subjective perspective. What do we feel? What do we feel we have to offer?

We may feel anger or a deep sadness. We may be experiencing a sense of loss that arises as we move away from one phase of our life into another. Sadness and grief, like anger, are normal, healthy emotions. Our challenge is to embrace our feelings and allow them to transform into something more healing. When we are able to be with all of our feelings, judgment is no longer the predominant way of seeing. We allow ourselves to be human. We familiarize ourselves with our inner voices that thrive in judging us. We turn down the volume when they criticize our failure to meet the cultural standards we believe we must fulfill. As we do when we forgive, we take a wide-angled view. We don't have to like our wrinkles, our loss of energy, but we can develop a new relationship with them, where they don't have power over us. We defuse their ability to make us feel worthless, undesirable or hopeless. Self-acceptance starts to replace fear and criticism. Compassion for ourselves arises. We don't have to be perfect. This is a shift from a cultural perspective to a personal one that is unique to who we are and our present experience.

We can never be wholly who we are if we define ourselves in terms of socio-cultural standards. We need to embark on the journey of self-discovery. Adopting culture-specific attitudes sidesteps the process that is needed to reveal our unique, authentic natures. Our Second Spring is often the time when we examine our personal belief systems. Take the time to consider what you believe versus what you've unconsciously internalized. It may be difficult to separate the two. Energetically, even holding an intention to question our attitudes and thoughts can powerfully influence our journey.

We may find we are angry at the cultural norms and pressures we feel we must fulfill or fit into. Maybe we will see how much we perpetuate the cultural concept of youth as a major means of shaping our lives. How much do I define myself by how young I look? Am I resisting this natural aging process? How do I accept myself? Can I accept all of what Second Spring brings? Can I use this as an opportunity for change? If we arrive at a level of self-acceptance, we will be able to be with ourselves with equanimity, tolerance and compassion. Where we are in life is OK. Who we are is just fine. This doesn't mean that we should not seek growth and healing in our lives.

Rather we become familiar with our inner worlds to honestly and courageously admit what we really hold as our truths and guiding beliefs. Do they serve us? Perhaps they once did, but do they work for us now? These are the forces that may be clouding our behaviour, attitudes and resistance to ourselves. They may prevent us from accepting who we are.

This is not a path for the faint-hearted. It takes courage, trust and perseverance to search for our personal inner truths. This may involve letting go of some long-held beliefs, but these energetic shifts have tremendous power to affect our physical well-being. In being emotionally honest, our Qi is allowed to flow smoothly. Obstructions become unblocked, energy moves freely. Blood can circulate evenly. The imbalances that give rise to many of our physical complaints will be addressed, influenced and ultimately ameliorated.

In cultures where menopausal women are accorded value, there is less likelihood of difficulties. Symptoms may be experienced but are interpreted differently. They are not seen as problems that require treatment. Rather, they may be viewed as indicators of the arrival of a new and respected phase of life. These are two very different energetic responses. The symptoms may be the same, but it is our response, our interpretation of them, that changes.

We have widened our perspective to include more than just our physical selves. We reflect on all Three Treasures—Jing, Qi and Shen. Healing is bringing harmony to each of these levels, our movement towards wholeness. This encompasses all aspects of who we are and our relationships. We shift from a perspective of separateness and autonomy to one of interconnection and interdependence. We take a holistic view of ourselves, not isolating our bodies from our emotions or from our spirit. As well, we enter into new relationships with others and our environment. Softening the grip of our separate protected ego, our hearts can then open to a greater context. There is room for everything, our imperfections and gifts, others' imperfections and gifts, and those of the environment.

Healing is a process of rediscovery in each moment. It is an awareness of what beliefs and attitudes support us in the movement towards wholeness and inner peace. In the present moment is where we may find our truth, our peace of mind. It is not in the past or in the future but in how we choose to live each moment. Moment by moment we trust the flow, trust our capacity to meet what arises, when it arises. We can be with the changing nature of aging, of illness, of health, of anger, of uncertainty, one moment at a time. As with labour, we only need to focus on this contraction that is arising, and then the next. We ride with them. We let go of their power over us. We are creating ourselves. We are giving birth to ourselves in this period of Second Spring.

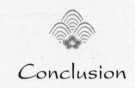

Conclusion

A daughter and her mother were walking in the mountains. Suddenly, the young girl fell, yelling, "AAhhh!" To her surprise, she heard a voice repeating, "AAhhh!" somewhere from the distant mountains. Curious, she yelled, "Who are you?" and was answered, "Who are you?" "I admire you!" she called, and the voice said, "I admire you!" Angered by this response, she yelled, "Coward!" The voice replied, "Coward!"

The girl looked at her mother and said, "What's going on?" Her mother smiled and said, "My daughter, pay attention." The mother called, "You are a champion!" and the voice answered, "You are a champion!" The girl was surprised, and did not understand. Her mother explained, "People call this 'echo,' but really this is life. It gives you back everything you say or do. Our life is simply a reflection of our actions and thoughts. Life will give you back everything you have given to it."

This story reminds us that our actions, words, thoughts and emotions have the power to shape who we are. There is a similar interrelatedness in Traditional Chinese Medicine. Our physical, emotional and spiritual health is a reflection of how we conduct our lives; how we take care of ourselves and what we believe about ourselves and the world. How we deal with our feelings, what we eat and drink, our physical activity, our sexual lives, our perception of who we are and the amount of rest we get profoundly affect our current stage of the feminine life cycle, and all subsequent phases. TCM acknowledges this interdependence by recognizing that our repressed anger is connected to our menstrual cramps; our habit of eating cold foods is linked to our breast lumps; our excessive exercise regime is associated with the loss of our Heavenly Water; our food cravings are connected to our infertility; our post-partum depression is linked to our loss of Blood after childbirth; our night sweats are associated with our use of oral contraceptives.

The basis of interrelatedness in TCM is Qi, the vital energy of the universe. Strong and free-flowing Qi in all its manifestations is what animates us and gives us health. Illness and symptoms are reflections of disharmony in the movement of Qi. Yin and Yang are the opposing yet complementary forces that, governed by the laws of the universe, sway between balance and imbalance. Balance in our bodies is directly related to the expression of our emotions, which are a manifestation of Qi. Feelings that are suppressed or excessive impact the smooth flow of Qi and the Liver, the Organ system responsible for the unobstructed movement of Qi in the body. The Liver also governs our menstrual cycle, so any blockages in the circulation of Qi will result in conditions during Heavenly Water that, if left untreated, can result in problems during our reproductive years. If we become ill or manifest symptoms during our fertile years and do not address the underlying causes, in Second Spring we will find ourselves enervated or ailing with the syndrome commonly referred to in the West as menopause.

Understanding our feelings and expressing them in healthy ways is critical to our feminine health. To do this we must re-examine our emotions and trust in our bodies and the wisdom within ourselves. Feeling confident comes about when we understand and accept ourselves, including our sexual needs. A satisfying sex life is important for our well-being, long life and spiritual journey. In connecting with our feelings and determining what is important to us, we are establishing new ways of being with ourselves and the changes that occur as we transition from one feminine phase to the next.

At the onset of Heavenly Water and through the first decade or so of its flow, we develop a new relationship with our bodies, and with our emotions. As we undergo the radical changes of puberty, we begin to redefine our relationship with ourselves.

During pregnancy we learn to let go. A natural series of biological changes has been set in motion that we have little ability to affect. As we relinquish the desire to control what is happening to our bodies, we also need to let go of our expectations for our identities and roles.

Golden Month is the time when we realize our unconditional love for our newborn. Our hearts open and we feel a deep connection with the inherent wisdom of our bodies and with mothers everywhere. As we marvel in the miracle of creation, we may experience ourselves within a larger context.

In Second Spring we move into acceptance. As we seek to

re-define ourselves against the cultural messages we've absorbed, we have the possibility to accept who we are and heal on a deep level, as we bring the Three Treasures, Jing (body), Qi (emotions) and Shen (spirit) into harmony.

Our journey from Heavenly Water to Second Spring is reflective of our healing journey into wholeness. It is a natural evolution from knowing ourselves on the level of the physical in Heavenly Water to connecting with the emotional aspects of ourselves in Ripening the Fruit. During Golden Month we develop a deep sense of connection to others. In Second Spring, we heal into wholeness as we integrate all aspects of ourselves.

I hope your journey through *Reflections of the Moon on Water* has provided you with a constructive introduction to women's health from a Traditional Chinese Medicine perspective. As a woman who has lived in both China and Canada, I hope that what I have learned about the phases and issues of a woman's life cycle has resonated with you and provided new perspectives, approaches and practices with which to move forward. Through preventative measures, it is we who have the greatest impact on our physical, emotional and spiritual health throughout the course of our lives. Let us reclaim our authority over our well-being and make it a priority. By incorporating Traditional Chinese Medicine in our lives, we have the opportunity to reconnect with the rhythms of nature and trust in the wisdom of who we are. We can restore our health, value ourselves for who we are and offer ourselves as a gift back to the world.

Acknowledgements

I would like to thank Marni Jackson, who, after interviewing me for her book *Pain*, urged me to write my own book, and then gave continuous encouragement as well as invaluable suggestions throughout the writing process. She introduced me to Anne Collins, publisher of Random House Canada, and senior editor Sarah Davies who, together with Louise Dennys, executive vice president of Random House of Canada, received my two-page proposal for the book with great enthusiasm. I am immensely grateful to them for their warmth, encouragement and belief in this book.

Thanks to Kanae Kinoshita, who not only helped me conceptualize and write this book but is also my best friend. I thank her for her time, her understanding, patience and care, for constantly challenging me, and for her ability to eloquently express on the page what was in my head and my heart.

To Stacey Cameron, my talented editor at Random House, who patiently helped shape the book and make it approachable without losing its essence. She has been truly exceptional!

To Linda Spalding and Michael Ondaatje, Linda Haynes, Devin Connell, Sara Rosenthal, Gabriella Martinelli and Ludwig Max Fischer, Barbara Minett, Diane Bald and Michael Budman, who read early drafts of the manuscript and gave me much needed encouragement, advice and support.

To Ann-Marie MacDonald, Susan Swan, Wende Cartwright, Alberta Noakes, Karen Minden, Tina Karpenchuk, Pauline Coutoure, Siamak Hariri, Sasha Rogers, Roya Mostaghim-Vaezi, Lorraine Segato, Naomi Duguid, Jeffrey Alford, Kathy Vieira, Leslie Lester, Liz Upchurch, Kate Hunter, Arlene Moscovitch, Ana Bodnar, Kristina Gordon, Debbi Haryett, Jessica Melchiorre, Denise Richard, Gunilla Robert, Michelle Metivier and Beverley Howell for their friendship, encouragement and support.

To David Bray, who helped me start practising TCM in Canada. He is a dear friend. His knowledge of TCM is unsurpassed, and he generously checked the medical information in this book. Whatever mistakes remain are mine alone.

To Yao Kemin, former president of Kunming Traditional Chinese Medicine Hospital, who inspired and helped me so much during my years under her leadership. I'd like to thank Cedric K.T. Cheung, president of the Chinese Medicine and Acupuncture Association of Canada and one of the first practitioners to introduce TCM to Canadians and pave the way for us who came later. I'd like to thank my TCM peers for their support and for spreading the practice of TCM in Canada: Denise Boutilier, Tsiao Yan Li, Wang Chao, Angela Warburton and Mary Wu.

I would like to thank Dr. Aref Vaezi, Dr. Harvey Schipper,

Dr. Carolyn DeMarco and Dr. Vincent DeMarco, doctors of Western medicine who have opened themselves to TCM and who support giving choice to their patients.

To Jennifer Shepherd, director of rights and contracts at Random House, for her belief in this book and for her patience and honesty. To Sharon Klein, my gifted publicist. To my dear friends Anka and Tom Czudec for taking the photo on the cover, and to Lynn Ryan for her support. To Kelly Hill for her wonderful jacket and page design. And to my dear old friend from Kunming, Hu Yaxong, for his lovely illustrations.

I'd like to thank my clinic staff Jin Nan, Gao Chao, Liu Yaokun, Xing Yuehua, Wei Hong and Shen Yilin who are all excellent TCM practiners, and especially Zhao (Lisa) Hong, who comes from the same city, graduated from the same TCM school and shares the same last name as me! She is my right-hand colleague, and without her I couldn't have written this book. I'd like to express my gratitude to my assistants, Hellen Hajikostantinov and Tao Liang—while I deal with my patients' stress, Hellen and Liang deal with mine.

I am grateful to all the women who shared their experiences and stories with me so that I might share them in this book. I hope they help other women in their healing journeys towards wholeness.

And finally, I'd like to thank my family: my parents, sisters and brother for their love and for always being there for me; my partner, Scott, for all his support, and for understanding this demanding life; and last, but certainly not least, my dear son, Zhao Zhao, who always gives his mother good advice and reminds her to look after herself.

Appendix

For updates and resources, visit www.xiaolanclinic.com.

MAJOR TCM AND ACUPUNCTURE ASSOCIATIONS IN NORTH AMERICA

If you are interested in finding a TCM practitioner or acupuncturist in your area, contact one of the following organizations for a recommendation:

CANADA

THE CHINESE MEDICINE AND ACUPUNCTURE ASSOCIATION OF CANADA
154 Wellington St.
London, ON
N6B 2K8
Tel: (519) 642–1970
Fax: (519) 642–2932
Website: www.cmaac.ca

**THE CANADIAN SOCIETY OF CHINESE MEDICINE AND
ACUPUNCTURE**
434 Dundas St. W., Suite 303
Toronto, ON
M5T 1G7
Tel/Fax: (416) 597-6769
Website: www.tcmcanada.org

BRITISH COLUMBIA

ACUPUNCTURE ASSOCIATION OF BRITISH COLUMBIA
411 Dunsmuir St.
Vancouver, BC
V6B 1X4
Tel: (604) 608–0608

**TRADITIONAL CHINESE MEDICINE ASSOCIATION
OF BRITISH COLUMBIA**
1200 Burrard St., Suite 801
Vancouver, BC
V6Z 2C7
Tel: (604) 602–9603

**UNITED ACUPUNCTURISTS ASSOCIATION
OF BRITISH COLUMBIA**
7031 Westminster Hwy, Suite 102A
Richmond, BC
V6X 1A3
Tel: (604) 821–1323

NOVA SCOTIA

**ACUPUNCTURE & NATUROPATHY ASSOCIATION
OF NOVA SCOTIA**
6066 Quinpool Rd.
Halifax, NS
B2L 1A1
Tel: (902) 492–8839

PRINCE EDWARD ISLAND

**ASSOCIATION OF REGISTERED ACUPUNCTURISTS
OF PRINCE EDWARD ISLAND**
44 Grafton St.
Charlottetown, PEI
C1A 1K5
Tel: (902) 628–1478

QUEBEC

ASSOCIATION D'ACUPUNCTURE DU QUÉBEC
441 Sainte-Hélène St., Suite 1
Longueuil, QC
J4K 3R3
Tel: (450) 679–0853 or (418) 623–9451
Fax: (450) 467–9213
Website: www.acupuncture-quebec.com

ORDRE PROFESSIONNEL DES ACUPUNCTEURS DU QUÉBEC
1600 Henri-Bourassa Blvd. W., Bureau 500
Montréal, QC
H3M 3E2
Tel: (514) 331–8870 or 1–800–474–5914

UNITED STATES

**NATIONAL CERTIFICATION COMMISSION FOR
ACUPUNCTURE AND ORIENTAL MEDICINE**
11 Canal Center Plaza, Suite 300
Alexandria, VA 22314
USA
Tel: (703) 548-9004
Fax: (703) 548-9079
Website: www.nccaom.org

Index